MISSED
CONCEPTIONS

MISSED CONCEPTIONS

HOW WE MAKE SENSE OF INFERTILITY

KAREN STOLLZNOW

BROADLEAF BOOKS
MINNEAPOLIS

MISSED CONCEPTIONS
How We Make Sense of Infertility

The names of some individuals have been changed to protect their privacy.

Cover image: Getty Images
Cover design: Alisha Lofgren

Print ISBN: 978-1-5064-8526-3
eBook ISBN: 978-1-5064-8527-0

Printed in Canada

This book is dedicated to Blade—always and forever.
It is also dedicated to others who discover that
the most natural thing in the world isn't.

CONTENTS

INTRODUCTION

Preconceptions

On August 7, 1908, Johann Veran discovered a small statue of a nude woman during an archaeological excavation at a site near Willendorf, a village in the Wachau Valley in Lower Austria. The figurine is faceless, her arms and feet are missing, but she has pendulous breasts resting on her swollen belly, curvaceous hips, and a pronounced vulva. The Woman of Willendorf, as she became known, was fashioned from limestone and tinted with red ocher pigment. She was carved during the Old Stone Age, a period of prehistory dating around 30,000 BCE. Archaeologists and historians offer a variety of interpretations of her meaning and use; perhaps she was a good-luck totem or a mother-goddess symbol, although her exaggerated childbearing features led anthropologists to suggest she was a fertility figurine. The Woman of Willendorf was made by a hunter-gatherer who may have carried the statue as a kind of Paleolithic fertility charm in the hopes of having children.

The Woman of Willendorf is one of the oldest known statues in the world, and as such, she is a touching testament to the age-old problem of infertility. Thousands of similar sculptures have been found at various archaeological sites around Europe and beyond. (They were originally called "Venus figurines," although they have no known association with the goddess Venus, whom they predate.)

Fertility figurines show that our ancestors also struggled with child-lessness, and that ancient societies searched for ways to solve this problem too. The figures represent the dream of parenthood for the people who carried them—a dream that still resonates today. They also reflect how we deal with infertility in the present. Perhaps a Paleolithic person carrying a fertility statue is no different from those today who, tens of thousands of years later, wear a fertility charm, pray to a saint, or visit the famed fertility statues at Ripley's Believe It or Not! museum in the belief that rubbing the statues' bellies will help them to conceive.

The struggle of infertility is a universal part of the human experience mentioned in the earliest writings. Recently, a four-thousand-year-old Assyrian tablet was discovered in the Kayseri province of Turkey, which is thought to be the first known mention of infertility. Written in the cuneiform script, the clay record is a prenuptial contract. It states that if the couple does not conceive within two years after the date of marriage, the wife should allow her husband to use a female slave to act as a surrogate. The slave would be freed after giving birth to the first male baby, ensuring that the family was not left without a child. We don't know how many people suffered infertility in the past, but history and folklore tell us that infertility has always been a problem. Fertility deities were worshipped in ancient Egypt, Greece, and Rome, and infertility is a central theme of creation stories, from Mesopotamian mythology to the book of Genesis in the Bible. Across cultures and time, the experiences of people who have faced fertility problems are widely discussed in early manuscripts, medical treatises, diaries, novels, poetry, plays, and songs.

Since the beginning of human history, we have tried to make sense of infertility. In the past, it was understood as punishment for sins, a curse, the result of an evil spell, or a test of faith. (Of course, some people still think this way.) Not being able to have children was at times believed to be a weakness, a moral failing, or a psychological disorder. Until infertility came to be seen as a medical condition, for many the arrival of a baby (or not) came down to chance. In ancient cultures, childless women were stigmatized. Women were believed to be responsible for fertility, so they were usually blamed when childbearing failed. It was a woman's social role to bear children and her duty as a wife; otherwise she faced serious repercussions. If her husband didn't take a concubine to bear his children, a woman who couldn't conceive might be divorced, shunned by society, or banished to a convent. In some extreme cases, she was exiled or even executed. Undoubtedly, infertility is still stigmatized today. Women with infertility are sometimes portrayed as abnormal, defective, or broken. They are victim-blamed—accused of being promiscuous, or too choosy when it comes to finding a partner, of prioritizing their careers, or of having "left it late" to have kids. Whether involuntarily childless or child-free by choice, women without children have often been cast as tragic figures regarded with disdain and pity. The good news is that these views are finally changing, and infertility is now being discussed more openly than any time before.

What exactly is infertility? Curiously, the contemporary definition isn't too different from the historical one. Infertility is defined as not being able to get pregnant after one year of having unprotected sex. Fertility is known to decline steadily with age, so for women over the age of thirty-five, infertility is defined as not being able to get pregnant after six months of trying. However, infertility isn't just about not being able to conceive. A key part of fertility is achieving a successful pregnancy, meaning one that results in the delivery of a healthy child. Women who are able to get pregnant but not to carry a baby to term may also be diagnosed with infertility. ("Pregnancy loss" refers to miscarriage, a fetal loss before twenty weeks of pregnancy, and also stillbirth, the loss of a baby any time from twenty weeks into the pregnancy through to the due date of birth.) Under the umbrella of infertility there are two main types. A woman who's never been able to get pregnant or achieve a live birth will be diagnosed as having primary infertility. Yet women who already have children can experience infertility too. A woman who has had at least one successful pregnancy in the past, but can't get pregnant again, will be diagnosed with secondary infertility.

The author of the ancient Assyrian tablet assumed that in the event of infertility the wife would be at fault, necessitating a surrogate. That the woman is always "to blame" is a stereotype that still exists today. Of course, infertility isn't just a woman's problem. Men can be infertile too. In fact, men and women are equally likely to have fertility problems. Statistically, about one-third of infertility cases can be attributed to women, while one-third can be attributed to men. The remaining third of cases may be caused by a combination of both male and female infertility. There are numerous reasons for infertility. Female infertility can be caused by a variety of medical conditions, including endometriosis or polycystic ovary syndrome (PCOS). Male infertility is generally related to issues with sperm, specifically their number, shape, or (in)ability to move. Various medications and drugs can also affect fertility in both men and women, as can risk factors for infertility, like older age. Frustratingly, in many cases the cause of infertility is simply unknown.

For individuals and couples, infertility is an adversity that has a profound effect on their emotions and experiences. It creates sadness, anger, frustration, and loneliness, and can cause depression and anxiety. Infertility is an incredibly difficult but surprisingly common part of the human experience. In the United States, about 12 percent of women have difficulty conceiving and carrying a child to term. One in six couples faces infertility, but after a woman turns thirty-five, one in three couples is infertile. Estimates suggest that more than one hundred million individuals suffer from infertility worldwide. It is considered a global public health problem, and it is on the rise. But being diagnosed with infertility doesn't mean that dreams of having a child must come to an end. It may take some time, but many couples who experience infertility will eventually be able to have a child. Some will do so on their own, while others will need help.

Humankind has contemplated the nature of infertility for thousands of years. Theologians, philosophers, and scientists have explored infertility, musing on its causes and effects, and offering many explanations and theories for its existence. Over time, infertility has been the domain of gods, clerics, oracles, folk healers, midwives, and doctors. Knowledge of infertility has progressed from being understood as a religious, magical, or moral issue to being recognized as a medical condition, and one that is treatable. Fertility treatments have advanced greatly in recent decades. Modern-day assisted reproductive technologies (ART) include intrauterine insemination (IUI) and in vitro fertilization (IVF). Since the birth of Louise Brown in 1978, the world's first "test-tube baby," IVF has become the gold-standard infertility treatment. To improve the outcomes of treatments, people can use donor eggs or sperm, or a surrogate (fortunately, a consensual one, rather than an enslaved person). The right kind of treatment depends on a variety of factors, such as the cause of infertility, how long the person or couple has been trying to conceive, their ages, and personal preferences. Over seven million women have used infertility services in the United States alone. Worldwide, ten million babies have been born via assisted technologies. Though the sobering truth is that fertility treatments don't always work, those who are trying to welcome a child into the home have more options now than ever before.

Missed Conceptions grew out of my own journey to conceive. When having a baby the old-fashioned way didn't work, I tried anything and everything I could think of to get pregnant. Along the way, I began to wonder how other cultures, and other eras, made sense of infertility. I devoured scriptures, manuscripts, collections of folklore, medical texts, science journals, books, online forums, and more—anything I could get my hands on that would help me understand this experience. The result is a book that situates my own story of trying to conceive within all of humankind's fertility struggles, past and present. My personal account is interspersed with vignettes and popular culture, myths and misconceptions, and hard science. I delve into history and mythology. I explore religion, faith, and spirituality. I test urban legends and old wives' tales, folk medicine and magic, and I try alternative therapies. Then I turn to modern science and medicine for answers. I shine a light on attitudes and beliefs about infertility as I immerse myself in the language and culture of those who experience it.

I didn't expect to have difficulty getting pregnant. No one ever does. After all, getting pregnant is supposed to be "the most natural thing in the world." But following a decade-long journey of missed conceptions, I learned that it isn't.

This is the story of my search to make sense of infertility.

1

BE FRUITFUL AND MULTIPLY

Do You Have Children?

I'd just reached my twenties when I was first asked this nosy question. It is considered rude to ask someone their age, how much they earn, or how they vote, but apparently it is completely acceptable to ask a stranger about their sex life and reproductive history.

This everyday question reveals the expectation that all women will get married and have children. Motherhood is seen as the traditional or supposedly "natural" role of women. Women are called the "gentler sex" and stereotyped as motherly and nurturing, with an inherent "maternal instinct." Society teaches girls that what it means to be a woman is to be a wife and a mother—to have babies. This gender role is learned at an early age when girls play with dollhouses and baby dolls. From childhood, the idea of marriage followed closely by having children is normalized in the way we talk. Like the nursery rhyme says, "First comes love. Then comes marriage. Then comes baby in the baby carriage." When a couple "settles down" and gets married, the next "normal" milestone in life is to "start a family." And social norms dictate that a couple must become parents in order to be considered a family. Friends and family ask, "When are you going to have children?" Mothers press for grandchildren with the demand, "When are you going to make me a grandmother?" Some would-be grandparents get pretty pushy about this too. In India, a couple sued their son and his wife for not giving them a grandchild after six years of marriage. The couple's lawyer said, "It is a dream of every parent to become a grandparent. They had been waiting for years to become grandparents."

Then strangers make small talk by asking, "Do you have children?"

Why do people want to have children anyway? Aside from the social pressure, there are many motives for wanting kids. Some people love children and want to create a family of their own. No one lives forever, and as we face our mortality, having a child can be a grasp at immortality. Having children can be a link to our past and our future. Some people experience an existential crisis in which they question their existence and purpose, and decide that a child might bring meaning and value to their life. Other people want to leave a legacy, to have an impact that transcends their own existence. Of course, plenty of people are child-free by circumstance or by choice, and yet they can still leave something behind. Isaac Newton never fathered a child, but his theories laid the groundwork for modern physics, and he became the "father of modern science." Jane Austen loved to give the characters in her books a happy ending, but her long and satisfying life did not include romantic love. While Austen didn't leave a family of her own behind, she did leave a literary legacy for readers to enjoy for centuries to come. But many people want a child who emerges in their own image, to embody their genes and carry on their bloodline.

Then there is the "biological instinct" to have children. This is the intense craving to be a mother that is felt from deep within and can't be reasoned or explained. Longing for a baby is often described as an uncontrollable "urge" to have kids. A woman who wants a baby is sometimes described as "broody" or "clucky," like a mother hen. Known in pop culture as "baby fever," this has long been immortalized in books, television, and movies. Baby fever can hit at a baby shower or strike at the sight of a rack of tiny baby shoes at the department store.

"Your nephew is so sweet, my uterus hurts," said Jamie Buchman in an episode of *Mad About You*.

Baby fever is associated with women, although men are not immune to this yearning for parenthood. Apparently, the urge decreases with age in women, and also for those who have become mothers already, but it actually *increases* for men as they grow older. The desire to become a parent is blamed on hormones and an evolutionary drive to pass on our genes. Surprisingly, there is no good evidence that the urge to have a child is innate. Scientists explain baby fever as a psychological and emotional reaction, which is influenced by social and cultural factors, not biological ones. Studies show that positive exposure to babies—cute ones who coo and smile and smell nice—makes people want to have kids. But not everyone catches baby fever; people who've had negative experiences with smelly toddlers and their temper tantrums might shy away from having their own. The drive might not be biological, but for those who catch baby fever, the phenomenon is no less real.

I'd experienced many bouts of baby fever myself, like the time I saw a pair of pink-sparkled shoes at the department store, although my urges were tempered in early adulthood by career goals, and later, I didn't act on them for financial and relationship reasons. That is, until the day I received a wake-up call. When I was thirty, I visited my gynecologist to have a Pap smear. I was lying on the examination table with my feet up in the stirrups when he asked casually, "Do you plan to have children?"

Definitely, I thought. *Someday.* I've always wanted to be a mother . . . eventually.

"Yes," I replied.

He leaped up from his swivel stool and loomed over me, brandishing a speculum in one gloved hand. "You're not a Hollywood celebrity who can afford expensive infertility treatments," he barked. "These are critical years for fertility. At your age, what are you waiting for?"

I was surprised by his brashness, but I had a good excuse. "I'm waiting to find a boyfriend."

In a newfound panic, I asked if there was some kind of test I could have to determine whether I was still fertile or not. But he informed me that women under the age of thirty-five should attempt to get pregnant for one full year before there is any need to have their fertility tested. "So you'd better find that boyfriend."

The biological urge may not exist, but the biological clock certainly does. When women realize their baby-making window is dwindling, some become frantic. The woman desperate to get married and have babies is a common trope; meanwhile, the man wants the baby-making sex but not the baby, and dodges commitment as long as he can.

After the doctor's lecture, my biological clock began ticking loudly. His words echoing in my ears, during a first date I blurted out to the poor guy, "I want to have a baby." I never heard from him again. Fair enough. But I needed a partner—doctor's orders.

Friends assured me that finding someone would happen when I least expected it, and it did. I finally found that boyfriend. (I also changed gynecologists.) That boyfriend, Matt, wanted to have a baby too (although I'd restrained myself from asking him about the delicate matter on our first date). After a short courtship, I moved from the San Francisco Bay Area to Denver to be with him and we got married. The next step was to have children and live happily ever after, right? But we weren't about to become one of those couples who have a honeymoon baby. From the very start, things weren't going to be easy for us. You see, my new husband required a vasectomy reversal before we could even try to conceive.

It Is Proper to Make People

One morning I was sitting in my favorite coffee shop, pondering my situation. I soon found myself staring at a mother reading to her daughter. The little girl had strawberry-blonde pigtails and a wide, toothless smile. I swear she was wearing those pink-sparkled baby shoes I'd seen at the department store. I felt an attack of baby fever come on as her mother caught my gaze. "Are you okay?" she asked.

I wasn't. But at least she didn't ask me if I had kids. With tears in my eyes, I found myself pouring my heart out to her. She touched my hand. "I'm June," she said. "And I believe we were meant to meet today."

June shared her story with me, which was remarkably similar to mine. Her husband had undergone a vasectomy in his previous relationship because he never expected to have children. The marriage ended in divorce, and he later married June. In this new marriage, they decided that they wanted to have children, so he had a vasectomy reversal. The adorable baby girl sitting on her lap was the result of this successful surgery. June recommended her surgeon, Dr. Davis, who ran a specialized clinic in San Antonio, Texas. His procedure was low-cost, and his patients had excellent pregnancy rates post-surgery. "He is doing God's work," she said, "by giving men another chance at having a family."

Following that fortuitous meeting with this kind stranger, I made an appointment for my husband and me to see Dr. Davis.

Having kids is not only a social expectation but a religious one too. On the very first page of the Bible, the command to procreate is given to Adam and Eve in the Garden of Eden: "And God blessed them, and said unto them, Be fruitful, and multiply, and replenish the earth, and subdue it: and have dominion over the fish of the sea, and over the fowl of the air, and over every living thing that moveth upon the earth" (Genesis 1:28 KJV). Similarly, the prophet Isaiah says, "For this is what the Lord says—he who created the heavens, he is God; he who fashioned and made the earth, he founded it; he did not create it to be empty, but formed it to be inhabited" (Isaiah 45:18 NIV). The encouragement to have kids is not limited to Judeo-Christian beliefs but extends to other world religions too. The Qur'an says, "O, Lord, grant us spouses and offspring who will be the comfort of our eyes" (25:74). Buddhism, Hinduism, and many other spiritual traditions also urge procreation and promote the importance of children and family.

The social expectation to have kids is not just a modern one. The need for children was essential across history. Reproduction was necessary to protect the economic stability of the family. With no welfare or pension in ancient times, offspring represented security in older age or times of illness, and the more kids, the better. Because of the high infant and child mortality rate, many children were needed so that some would survive into adulthood. Having kids was also crucial to safeguard the strength of society and ensure the continuation of the species. That producing children, and many of them, was seen as the moral and right thing to do is documented in the earliest writings. In an ancient Egyptian text, the scribe Any, who worked in the court of Nefertari, says to his son, "It is proper to make people. Happy the man whose people are many."

Sexist gender roles existed in ancient societies too. Men and women were expected to conform to social and family roles in which it was a woman's duty to bear children. For much of history, women had few rights or liberties, but they were valued for their role as child-bearers. Young men were counseled to prioritize fertility above other womanly attributes and were required to marry a "hot-limbed" woman. This expression was the ancient equivalent of *childbearing hips*, referring to a fertile and fruitful woman who was capable of bearing many children. In those days, fertility was the measure of womanhood. A "real" wife and "proper" woman was, by definition, one who bore children to continue her husband's lineage. A good wife gave her husband some, if not many, offspring. Throughout history, many women spent most of their adult years pregnant. In ancient Greece, a woman only entered full woman-hood upon delivery of a child, and preferably a son. Historically, boys were preferred for their labor power and inheritance rights and because they would carry on the family name, while they didn't require a dowry upon marriage. This bias appears in the earliest writings too. An ancient Vedic text reads, "O woe is the woman who does not carry out the provided role of a mother [birth of sons]. O woe the unmarried, woe the childless, woe the mother of daughters, the widow."

This kind of pronatalism (the push to have lots of kids) was popular throughout history, especially during times of falling birth rates. In some societies, not having children was even punished. In ancient Rome, the birth rate was low due to husbands who were absent on military campaigns, the growing use of birth control, and the prevalence of infanticide and child exposure (particularly of newborn girls, because parents wanted boys). To combat the declining birth rate, Caesar Augustus introduced laws that made celibacy illegal and penalized bachelors and childless couples. Abortion was criminalized and infanticide made a capital offense. On the other hand, fertility was rewarded. Family allowances were given for having children, and mothers had the honor of wearing special clothing to show their status. In the end, these measures failed. Childlessness was widespread and has been blamed, in part, for the collapse of the Roman Empire.

Having children was also encouraged in the wake of the Black Death, which devastated the population of Europe during the Middle Ages. To persuade people to repopulate, clergy encouraged their congregations to "Be fruitful, and multiply." The global population was further diminished by low life expectancy and high mortality rates due to disease, war, and later marriage, which restricted a couple's fertile years. Birth rates remained low for hundreds of years after the bubonic plague. In response, *Aristotle's Masterpiece* (which was not written by Aristotle, nor really a masterpiece) emerged with a pronatalist agenda, because the world was apparently "being weakened by underpopulation." This was an early sex manual, dealing variously with "the use and actions of the genitals," "signs of conception," and "signs of barrenness." It was bawdy and irreverent, giving recommendations like, "If she is ugly, the advice is: do it in the dark." A seventeenth-century version of *The Joy of Sex*, the book was considered pornographic and was banned many times, although it remained a bestseller until the early twentieth century.

Pronatalism has an ugly side. During World War II, eugenics laws were introduced in both Nazi Germany and Fascist Italy. Dictator Benito Mussolini envisioned an Italian Empire to rival the Romans. Under his regime, the "Battle for Births" encouraged couples to have five children per family. Wartime propaganda associated motherhood, children, and family with national greatness (but only if they were white). When Adolf Hitler became the German chancellor, he urged women to have more babies to "provide soldiers for the next wars." To foster traditional families in the Third Reich, allowances were given to men whose wives gave up working, couples received payments for having children, and mothers who had four or more kids were awarded the "Mother's Cross" medal. But this honor only applied to "Aryan" women. Those considered "undesirable" and "inferior," such as Jews, Communists, and women with disabilities, were instead sterilized to prevent them from producing "degenerate" children.

With the renewed domesticity of women post-war, there was an increase in birth rates known as the "baby boom." The children of the era are well known as the "baby boomers." But today it's said that we're in the midst of a baby *bust*, because people in

Western countries are choosing to have fewer children. While many are concerned about global overpopulation and its impact, this downward trend in fertility has created a modern pronatalism movement. Just like in ancient Rome, pronatalist policies have been introduced in Sweden, Japan, Hungary, and other countries, and incentives offered to encourage more people to have children. Some countries impose penalties or taxes on those without children. (In contrast, China introduced a one-child policy in 1980, designed as a temporary measure to curb the country's population growth. The strategy was abandoned in 2016, when the nation's fertility fell well below the replacement level and China faced mounting pressures associated with low fertility.)

The idea of collapsing fertility rates has been explored in works of fiction. In the dystopian book and television series *The Handmaid's Tale*, worldwide infertility has led to the enslavement of fertile women. This group includes divorcées, single or unmarried mothers, lesbians, and non-Christians who are branded "fallen women." In a climate of religious fanaticism, these women, called Handmaids, are assigned to the homes of the ruling elite, where they must submit to ritualized rape by their male masters, to be impregnated and bear children for them.

In the West, higher fertility rates are often tied to religiosity. The creation mandate "Be fruitful and multiply" is still practiced by some branches of Christianity, particularly Catholics, Mormons, and the Amish. The Amish are among the fastest growing populations in the world. Much higher than the stereotypical average of 2.5 kids per family, a typical Amish woman has given birth to 7.1 children.

But I would've been happy with just one.

Chief of Staff

Matt lay on the operating table while the surgical team stood over him, ready to perform his reverse vasectomy. I had been allowed to stay in the room to watch the procedure, so I stood nervously in the background, dressed in a blue surgical gown, cap, and booties. Upon arrival we were surprised to discover that this wasn't a typical medical clinic, but a Christian mission. Wearing bandana scrub caps saying "God Bless America" and adorned with American flags, the team hung their heads as Dr. Davis recited a prayer. "Dear Lord, we pray that you watch over us during this surgery. We ask that this vasectomy reversal be successful so that Matthew can father more of your children. In Jesus's name. Amen."

"Amen," the team responded in unison.

Matt had been given a local anesthetic only, so he was awake during the procedure. Feeling anxious and awkward, he searched for somewhere to look. There was a cross hanging on the wall at his feet and a portrait of the Virgin Mary and child. Matt raised his eyes above and noticed there was another painting on the wall behind him. The artwork showed an operating room, with medical staff performing surgery on a patient, while Jesus guided the surgeon's hands. The caption read: "Chief of Staff." Matt stifled a laugh and tried to hold still as the surgeon began performing the delicate microsurgery.

A vasectomy is a surgical procedure for male sterilization when a man decides he doesn't want any (more) children. At the time of Matt's reversal, a friend with three sons was undergoing a vasectomy because, in his words, "If I merely sneeze on my wife I get her pregnant." Vasectomy is known colloquially (and to men, cringingly) as "the snip," because it involves cutting the vas deferens, the tube that carries a man's sperm from his testicles to his urethra. Men who have vasectomies still make sperm, but cutting the vas deferens blocks the sperm from getting to his semen when he ejaculates, to prevent pregnancy. The first recorded vasectomy was performed in 1823, when British surgeon Sir Ashley Cooper experimented on his pet dog. Apparently the procedure had no adverse effects on the canine's sex life.

Vasectomies weren't performed on humans until the 1900s, although they weren't done for sterilization purposes but with the intention of shrinking enlarged prostate glands and removing bladder stones. The operation had no such benefits; however, vasectomy soon became a weapon of the eugenics movement in the United States. The procedures were used to sterilize "undesirables" and "social parasites," including habitual criminals and "chronic inebriates, imbeciles, perverts and paupers." They were also used (unsuccessfully) to cure "excessive masturbation" in youths. Involuntary vasectomy has been prohibited since the 1960s, but not before tens of thousands of men were made infertile against their wishes.

Nowadays, vasectomies are regarded as a method of consensual birth control, although they are not very popular. Only 2.2 percent of the world's men have had vasectomies. They are cheaper, faster, safer, and more reliable than female sterilization, although 18.9 percent of women shoulder the responsibility for contraception by undergoing tubal ligation. Some men eschew vasectomies because they're concerned about the pain and fearful that the procedure will damage their sexual organs or affect their sexual performance. In the past, the opposite was thought to be true. During the "roaring twenties," it was popularly believed that having a vasectomy was the fountain of youth that could restore general vigor and sexual potency. This idea was based on experiments physiologist Eugen Steinach conducted on senile rats that were supposedly "rejuvenated" by the treatment. Vasectomies became so fashionable that his name became a verb. Many prominent men were "Steinached," including Sigmund Freud, who underwent the procedure when he was sixty-seven years old, hoping it would boost his waning sex drive. William Butler Yeats had one of these so-called therapeutic vasectomies at the age of sixty-nine, gushing that it gave him a "second puberty" and "revived [his] creative power." Unlike castration, in which the testes are removed, vasectomies do not affect the production of sperm or testosterone. And we have no data to show that vasectomies reduce a man's libido in any way, nor that they boost his sex drive, energy, or intelligence.

Vasectomies are largely successful, but occasionally they don't work. A vasectomy failure (pregnancy) can happen when a couple has unprotected sex too soon, before the sperm can clear out of the semen. Sometimes the procedure does not fully block the vas deferens and needs to be redone. In rare cases of recanalization, the vas deferens grows back and creates a new connection, causing the vasectomy to reverse itself. Some men later regret their decision to have a vasectomy because life circumstances change. A couple may decide they now want children (or more children), or a man decides he wants children from a new marriage, which is what happened in my case. Vasectomies are permanent unless they are reversed. The first "repair" was done in 1907 in an attempt to reverse an accidental vasectomy that occurred during a hernia operation. Of the 10 percent of men who undergo a vasectomy, a further 10 percent will choose to undergo a reverse vasectomy. A reversal reattaches the tubes to allow them to carry sperm from the testicles to the semen. Following successful surgery, sperm are present in the semen again and the man may be able to get his partner pregnant. However, reversals are not as affordable as vasectomies. Reverse surgery is more complicated than vasectomy, and there is no guarantee it will work. Matt had his vasectomy over ten years ago, and the longer a man waits to reverse the procedure, the less likely it is he'll be able to father children.

The operating room fell silent as Dr. Davis sat at his desk peering into a microscope. When he finally looked up again, he wore a smile on his face. "We have sperm!" he announced to applause.

During the reversal, the vas deferens is checked for sperm. If there are none, there is likely a blockage. If sperm are present, then the two ends of the vas deferens can be put back together and the surgery will likely be successful.

"How do you tell the urethra apart from the testicles?" the doctor asked. "There's a vas deferens between them!" His joke was met with groans.

"Let's get you sewn back up again," he said.

Matt wasn't in any pain, but he grimaced as he felt the pressure and tugging from the stitching. Some time later, looking a little green, he hobbled out of the operating room. The whole procedure had taken less than two hours.

As we were leaving, we stopped to take a look at the waiting room walls, which were covered with photographs of babies born from successful vasectomy reversals. "Children are a gift from God," said Dr. Davis.

Having finished his surgeries for the day, he accompanied us back to our car. On the way, he explained his Christian mission.

He believed it was his calling to provide vasectomy reversals so that couples could have children. Then he handed us a copy of the Bible. "I'm doing God's work," he told us. Apparently God's work paid a lot, we thought, as he stepped into his luxury car. "May the Lord bless you in your journey to start a family."

That evening we explored San Antonio and went for a romantic stroll along the famous River Walk. Well, it would've been romantic if Matt wasn't feeling squeamish because he'd just had a reverse vasectomy. We were anxious to test out the reversal, but we had been told to abstain from intercourse for two weeks following the procedure. Having sex too early after a reverse vasectomy can be painful for the man. There is also the potential for serious complications, such as ruptures and infections. We were advised to take things slowly. There was plenty of time for baby-making.

Testicular Fortitude

Three months after the surgery we received a phone call from the clinic. It was the surgical nurse following up to see how we were both doing post-operation. "Are you pregnant yet?" she asked up front.

"Not yet," I replied.

"That's normal," she said. "It can take months for sperm to appear in the semen again."

Months? I wish I'd known that earlier, I thought. I'd read glowing testimonials on the clinic's website bragging of couples getting pregnant almost immediately after a reversal, even if the vasectomy had been performed many years before.

"We'll keep trying," I assured the nurse.

"Good luck," she said. "We look forward to getting a baby picture for our walls!"

Women are born with all the eggs they'll ever have, although men aren't born with ready-made sperm. Boys start producing spermatozoa (or sperm, for short) at the onset of puberty. This usually begins at around ten or twelve years old, although some start a little sooner while others start a little later. Sperm begin developing in the testicles. The swimmers then gather in a long, coiled tube called the epididymis before mixing with semen just prior to ejaculation. The male body is constantly at work producing sperm, making several million sperm per day. Ideally, a man makes about 1,500 every second. The average sperm lives only a few weeks inside a man's body, and in a man who hasn't had a vasectomy, about 250 million sperm are released with each ejaculation. If sperm aren't ejaculated, the body absorbs them, which is what happens to men who've had vasectomies. In those who haven't had the snip, sperm might also be released during wet dreams.

As the nurse revealed, it can take months for a reverse vasectomy to work. Men who've had vasectomies continue to make sperm, although it can take a while to show up in their semen again after a reversal. Sperm may appear in the semen within a few weeks of surgery, but it may take up to a year or even longer. Sperm quality can take time to improve too, because it takes several months for the testicles to make new sperm. New sperm are being produced all the time, but they need about two to three months to fully mature. Doctors don't tell you that it can be difficult to get pregnant after a reverse vasectomy. Conceiving after a reversal usually takes a couple from six months to a year, if it ever happens at all. The true rate of pregnancy after vasectomy reversal can range from 30 to

70 percent. The chances of a successful reversal may be lower if it's been over ten years since the vasectomy. You can't always trust the glowing testimonials.

Those baby pictures were going to take a little longer than we'd thought.

God Opened Her Womb

It had now been six months since the reversal, but we hadn't had any luck yet on the baby front. I decided to call the clinic to speak directly with Dr. Davis for any advice he might have.

"This is normal," he told me. "It can take a while for sperm to appear in the semen again."

"That's what the nurse said months ago," I replied. I was a little disappointed to hear the same thing again.

"Do you still have that Bible I gave you?"

"Er . . . yes," I said as I mentally searched my house for the book. I knew I had it somewhere.

"Then read the story of Sarah and Abraham in the book of Genesis," he said. "They went through a test of faith too. Be patient and it will happen."

I sighed. "It's hard to be patient when my biological clock is ticking loudly."

"I know," he said. "But God *will* open your womb . . . when the time is right."

I rummaged through my house, but I couldn't find the book. I eventually checked the suitcase I'd taken to San Antonio all those months ago, and there it was, still safely zipped up in the front pocket. I read the story of Sarah and Abraham, and it sent me down a rabbit hole.

Despite the divine directive to be fruitful and multiply, barrenness is a common theme in the Bible. Most familiar are the narratives of Sarah, Rebekah, and Rachel, the "matriarchs" of Israel in the Old Testament. In Sarah's story, the one the doctor suggested I read, God said to her husband, Abraham, "'Look up at the sky and count the stars—if indeed you can count them. . . . So shall your offspring be'" (Genesis 15:5 NIV). God promised the couple a son, but they laughed it off because they were too old to have children. Nevertheless, when Abraham was a centenarian and Sarah ninety years old, she miraculously gave birth to a son, Isaac. But then Isaac and his wife, Rebekah, also struggled to have children. After many years of marriage, Rebekah had still not given birth and was believed to be barren. For decades, the couple prayed fervently for a child, and God eventually answered their prayers. When Isaac was sixty, they were blessed with twin sons, Esau and Jacob (Genesis 25:26).

But the family was to suffer three generations of infertility. Jacob would also have difficulty conceiving with his preferred wife, Rachel. (Yes, he was married to two women, and sisters at that.) In the saga of Rachel and Leah, the narrator says, "When God saw that Leah was unloved, he opened her womb," and over time she gave birth to seven children, "but Rachel was barren" (Genesis 29:31 NKJV). In competition with each other for the affections of their husband, they offered Jacob their handmaids, Zilpah and Bilhah, as concubines, who both bore him more sons. (In *The Handmaid's Tale*, mentioned above, the story is based on an extremist interpretation of the biblical account of Bilhah, the slave surrogate.) In the ancient Near East, it was the custom for a man to conceive children with an enslaved woman if his marriage proved to be infertile. Just like the four-thousand-year-old marriage contract mentioned in the introduction, wives were expected to allow their husbands to father children with enslaved women if the couple couldn't conceive (making the presumption that *she* was the infertile party). Any children born then belonged to the married couple. This practice may sound strange, but it was somewhat comparable to modern-day surrogacy (although enslaved women were subjected to inequity and abuse and couldn't consent to pregnancy in the way that most modern surrogates do). Back to the Bible: Rachel prayed desperately for years to have a child of her own. "Then God remembered Rachel, and God listened to her and opened her womb" (Genesis 30:22 NKJV). She conceived and bore a son, Joseph. Rachel then prayed for another child and gave birth to a second son, Benjamin, although tragically, she died during childbirth.

Infertility also features prominently in other creation stories, including Mesopotamian mythology. The Atrahasis epic, recorded in the Akkadian language on clay tablets, tells of a primeval flood story that predates the narrative of Noah's ark and the biblical flood. The epic was written in the seventeenth century BCE, although the tale itself is much older, having been passed down through oral tradition. According to the story, the gods were concerned about human overpopulation, so they unleashed a devastating flood to destroy human life. Only a wise and kindly man named Atrahasis was secretly warned of the coming flood by the god Enki, who instructed the man to build an ark to save himself. Atrahasis heeded the words of the god, loaded two of every kind of animal into the ark, and so preserved life on earth. When the other gods discovered that a human had survived the flood, they were angry. As a solution to avoid excess reproduction in the future, they resolved to create humans who were less fertile. The mother goddess Ninmah took a lump of clay and "fashioned a woman who could not give birth." From that point on, there would be women who could give birth, but also those who could not. She became known as *la ālittu*, "a woman who does not bear."

According to the Hebrew Scriptures, fertility was a blessing, while childlessness was seen as a curse or punishment for sin. In Hosea 9:14 NIV, God punishes the Israelites' idolatry with the threat of "wombs that miscarry and breasts that are dry." Barrenness was God's will. In Rachel's story, she cried to her husband, "Give me children, or I'll die!" Jacob replied, "Am I God? He's the one who has kept you from having children!" (Genesis 30:1–2 NLT). Fertility was a gift from God, "the fruit of the womb a reward" (Psalm 127:3 NRSV). When Rachel finally gave birth to a son, she declared, "God has taken away my disgrace" (Genesis 30:23 NIV), her "disgrace" being her barrenness. Fertility was also God's will, and pregnancy a result of divine intervention. God had to "open the womb" for Rachel to conceive. As the Talmud says, "The key of the womb is in the hands of the Lord" (Taanit 2a). But all births stopped when a woman's "womb was closed," like a door.

Throughout the Bible, women who suffer infertility are described as "barren" (*'aqar* in Hebrew). Yet some of these women, including the matriarchs, are not truly barren in the sense of biologically incapable of bearing children, because they eventually *do* conceive and give birth. Barrenness is also defined against the backdrop of actually *wanting* to have children. In the stories of other biblical women who have no offspring, including Jacob and Leah's daughter Dinah, Queen Esther, the prophet Miriam, and Mary Magdalene, they are never labeled as "barren," because (to the best of our knowledge) they never wanted children in the first place.

In the Bible, barrenness is often a literary device that foretells the miraculous birth of a divinely chosen leader. In the book of Luke, it was part of God's plan that the "barren" Elizabeth gave birth to St. John the Baptist in her old age. When the once-barren Sarah, Rebekah, and Rachel became the mothers of Isaac, Jacob, and Joseph respectively, God's promise to Abraham was fulfilled, and he became the father of the Jewish people. Barrenness also served as a lesson to keep the faith. Manoah's wife (Judges 13:2) and Hannah (1 Samuel 1) are also described as "barren," although through their persistent prayer and faith in God they are eventually "remembered" and rewarded with children. However, God didn't remember to open the wombs of all barren women. In the second book of Samuel, Michal, the younger daughter of King Saul and the first wife of David, "had no children to the day of her death" (2 Samuel 6:23 NIV).

Old Testament "fire and brimstone" aside, I found it strangely comforting to read about couples facing barrenness in the Bible. It made me feel less alone. I was inspired by the faith and courage of these women in the face of infertility, giving me confidence that I could face it too. It gave me hope to learn about the stories of women who believed they were barren, only to go on to have children. I thought it was touching that Sarah, a woman who was "barren" for most of her life, would eventually become the mother of an entire nation, with descendants as numerous as the stars of the sky.

But I certainly couldn't wait until *I* was ninety years old to have a baby!

Keeping the Faith

More months went by without success. It had now been nine months since the vasectomy reversal. *I could've had a baby in this time*, I thought wryly. But at my age and having tried for less than a year, according to my former gynecologist it was still too early for me to investigate my own fertility. So I emailed Dr. Davis. "Is there anything else we can do?" I asked him.

"Keep the faith," he wrote. "God has a plan for you. Pray."

Back at my local coffee shop one morning, I bumped into June again. Her daughter was growing up fast. A babe in arms when I'd last seen her, she was now walking and exploring the world around her. Her strawberry-blonde hair was longer now, and she was even uttering a few words. Her developments called to my attention the passage of time.

Over lattes I brought June up to speed on my situation. "I just don't know what to do from here."

"I think we were meant to meet again," June said. "Let me show you something that helped me." She scribbled down an address on a napkin and handed it to me. "Meet me here tonight at seven, and bring your husband along too." It all sounded rather mysterious.

"Perhaps she sells Amway?" suggested Matt as we drove to the place at the appointed time.

We arrived at the address written on the napkin. It was a church. "At least it's not Amway," quipped Matt.

We considered leaving—we weren't in the mood for proselytizing. But we *were* a little curious. We went inside the church and spotted June with her husband and daughter. She dashed over to greet us. "I'm so glad you could make it for the healing prayer tonight," she said.

Matt and I exchanged a furtive glance with each other and then glanced at the door . . .

In the Scriptures, several "barren" women are healed miraculously. As we've seen, God "remembered" Sarah, Rebekah, Rachel, and others, opening their wombs so they could bear children after many years of barrenness. In the apocryphal First Gospel of James (not to be confused with the New Testament book of James), God also healed Joachim and Anne of their infertility. Another older couple, they had prayed for a child throughout their marriage, and their neighbors scorned them for being childless. In desperation, Joachim withdrew to the desert to fast and pray for a time, while Anne prayed under a laurel tree. (One would think being apart would make pregnancy even more difficult!) Hearing their prayers, the angel Gabriel visited them separately and promised that, despite their advanced age, they would conceive a daughter. Their test of faith was rewarded. When she was eighty years old, Anne bore a child, Mary, who would become the mother of Jesus Christ. To this day, people experiencing infertility pray for St. Anne to intervene, because she is the patron saint of childless couples. (Apparently she can also help people find lost objects.)

Since ancient times, people have been making pilgrimages to holy sites, hoping to be healed of their infertility. Rachel's Tomb in Bethlehem, near Jerusalem, is believed to be the place the matriarch was buried after dying in childbirth and is a popular destination for modern women facing infertility. Pilgrims wrap a red string around the tomb seven times, which is then worn across the hips as a fertility charm. Around the world are shrines built to St. Anne, some containing alleged holy relics, like strands of her hair or bone fragments. Childless couples flock to these sanctuaries to petition her for a child. Others turn to St. Anne's daughter, Mary, to overcome their infertility. According to the Bible, the angel Gabriel visited Mary too, telling her, "You will conceive in your womb and bear a son, and you shall call his name Jesus" (Luke 1:31 ESV). As what Roman Catholics and others call an "immaculate conception," the Virgin Mary's pregnancy was a miracle, and people still turn to her, hoping for a miracle of their own. In Naples, Italy, there is a chair said to have been owned by St. Mary Frances of the Five Wounds of Jesus. People travel from far and wide to sit in the "miracle chair," later claiming to be blessed with a baby. Many Catholic saints are devoted to infertility, St. Agnes, St. Collette, and St. Rita among them. Praying to these saints to heal infertility or praying to God for intervention is based in the Old Testament doctrine that barrenness was a curse, a punishment for sins, or the result of a lack of faith.

There was plenty of healing in the New Testament too. Jesus and his apostles performed dozens of miraculous cures, although they were busy healing leprosy, casting out demons, and raising people from the dead, rather than curing barrenness. The Epistle of James mentions faith healing: "Is anyone among you sick? Let them call the elders of the church to pray over them and anoint them with oil in the name of the Lord. And the prayer offered in faith will make the sick person well" (5:14–15 NIV). In the past, kings were thought to have the ability to heal too, because they were appointed by God and anointed with holy oil. The "royal touch" of a monarch was believed to have miraculous powers to cure diseases, including barrenness. During the eleventh century, Edward the Confessor washed the neck of a "scrofulous woman" who was also barren. It was said that her scrofula (a type of tuberculosis) disappeared immediately and she later gave birth to twins. Some people believe that God and Jesus still heal supernaturally. Healing with hands-on prayer is a practice in modern Christianity, particularly in Pentecostal and charismatic churches, like the one June led me to. Believers claim faith healing can cure anything from cancer to infertility.

"Do you want to be healed of your infertility?" asked the minister.

Matt and I looked at each other. *What have we got to lose?* I thought. "Yes," we both replied.

A group of people encircled us. They laid their hands on our shoulders and muttered quiet prayers. The minister produced a little glass bottle of oil, dabbed some on his thumb, and then used it to draw a cross on our foreheads. "I anoint you with this oil in the name of the Holy Spirit," he said. He placed the palm of his hand on my forehead. "Lord Jesus, you know that this marriage has not yet been blessed with a child and how much they desire this gift."

"Praise Jesus!" shrieked one of the people in the circle.

"We come to you to ask that you heal this couple's infertility," the minister continued. "Hear our plea, Lord, and grant them a child from their love."

The praying around us grew louder.

"We know that through you, all things are possible," said the minister, as he pressed harder against my forehead. "In the name of the Father, and of the Son, and of the Holy Spirit. Amen!"

"Amen!" cried the group.

The minister pushed hard against my forehead, and I fell backward into the arms of the people standing behind me.

Afterward, I felt overwhelmed and exhausted by the experience. Not having grown up in a particularly religious household, I found faith healing very strange. I felt awkward being anointed with oil and prayed over in front of an audience, like I was part of a tent revival or onstage at a televangelist show. I noted that instead of "laying hands" on me, the minister had *pushed* me.

But for all the bizarreness of the event, I appreciated that they were trying to help. It also gave me a sense of hope.

"Never give up," said June as she gave me a farewell hug. "There's always hope."

Many people, when they experience difficulties getting pregnant, turn to religion to find hope and meaning in their suffering. Giving themselves over to a "higher power" can give comfort and strength and help them cope. Being reminded that "God has a plan for you" and to "keep the faith" can be reassuring. Faith can be understood as trust in God, but it can also mean confidence and optimism. Religious messages like these can be helpful, but they can also be harmful.

Some people take a fatalistic approach to fertility, that pregnancy is either "God's will" or "not meant to be." Even today, for many, fertility is a matter of faith. Some say people with infertility can't get pregnant because they have sin in their lives or they need to have a better relationship with God. But of course, there are many couples who pray, read the Scriptures, attend worship services, and even receive faith healing but who nevertheless remain unable to conceive. This doesn't mean they are cursed, sinful, or lacking in faith. Cruelly, some people with infertility are told God doesn't want them to become parents, or God thinks they would be bad parents. Such statements made in the name of religion are ignorant, judgmental, and victim-blaming. In the end, it doesn't matter what we believe or don't believe—infertility can affect anyone.

For Matt and me, before we could be healed of infertility, perhaps we needed to find out whether we were actually infertile.

Maybe we just needed to give it more time.

2

THE MOST NATURAL THING IN THE WORLD

The Birds and the Bees

"How's the baby-making going?" asked my friend Kate with a nudge and a wink. We were shopping for an upcoming baby shower for a mutual acquaintance.

"Not as successfully as it's going for others," I said with a nod to the baby gifts we carried, and to the throng of pregnant women in the store. Now that I was trying to have a baby, it seemed like everyone else around me was already pregnant. It reminded me of the frequency illusion of when you buy a new car and then suddenly see the same make or color everywhere.

"But it's fun trying to get pregnant, isn't it?" Kate giggled.

Sometimes, I thought.

At times, sex with the intention of making a baby loses its spontaneity and can feel like a chore. "Bedroom burnout," they call it. Trying to conceive is also stressful because of the pressure to succeed, especially the more you fail. Sex for procreation can bring about a whole new level of performance anxiety.

Kate picked up a greeting card and handed it to me. It said, "Congratulations! It's a girl!" and pictured a flying stork delivering a newborn baby wrapped up safely in a cozy pink bundle. "Don't worry," she said. "One day the stork will be delivering *your* bundle of joy!"

Newborn babies are often depicted with an unlikely creature: a long-legged, sharp-beaked stork. The image of this bird, usually dangling a cloth bundle in its beak, is ubiquitous on greeting cards and baby clothes. The legend tells that storks find babies in caves or marshes and carry them to households in a bundle held in their beak. But why storks? White storks live in colonies close to people, who witness the birds' nesting behavior and associate them with parenting and fertility. The myth most likely originated in medieval Europe, when couples were married during the summer solstice at festivals honoring fertility. Coincidentally, storks would start their annual migration south at this time, to spend the winter months in the warmer African climate. They returned to Europe the following spring for their breeding season, exactly nine months later, just when all the newlyweds were giving birth to their honeymoon babies. The myth was popularized in the nineteenth century by Hans Christian Andersen's short story "The Storks." In this tale, the birds plucked dreaming babies from ponds and lakes to deliver them to deserving families. But the story has a forgotten, dark underside. Families with naughty children received a dead baby from the stork as punishment.

The stork story became a traditional response to the awkward question, asked by kids, "Where do babies come from?" But it wasn't the only euphemistic story for explaining reproduction to curious children considered too young for "the talk" about sex or "the birds and the bees." For hundreds of years, folklore told that babies were also brought by other animals, like owls, foxes, ravens, and crows. Some legends say babies came from fairies, water sprites, or wild women of the forest. In Germany, there was the legend of Der Kindlbringer, the bringer of babies to new parents. He dressed like a harlequin and carried a bundle of babies in a bunting or on his back. Babies might also be discovered under a gooseberry bush or in a lime tree. The legend that babies were found in a cabbage patch gave rise to the 1980s phenomenon of Cabbage Patch Kids. These cloth dolls with plastic faces came with a birth certificate and adoption papers. I had one when I was a kid. She was a chubby-faced girl with blonde braids and freckles; her birth certificate introduced her as Meghan May.

Today, these legends seem quaint and old-fashioned, but they're not just relics of the prudish Victorian era. Some mothers and fathers continue to tell them, alongside stories of Santa Claus and the tooth fairy. Other parents talk quite literally about "the birds and the bees," relying on imagery of bees pollinating and eggs hatching to avoid a more technical explanation of sexual intercourse, although the vague connection between human sexuality and birds and bees can cause confusion for kids. This is satirized in an episode of the TV show *The Simpsons* when ten-year-old Bart Simpson says to his friend Milhouse, "The sun is out, birds are singing. The bees are trying to have sex with them, as is my understanding."

Papa Don't Preach

One day at school when I was about eight years old, I was playing with a group of friends during lunchtime. We carefully avoided a group of boys nearby because, we were sure, they would infect us with "cooties" if they touched us. All of a sudden, the loathsome Lucas Wright broke free of the group, swaggered over to me, and planted a kiss directly on my lips! I was humiliated. The boys burst into laughter, but we girls were utterly horrified. One girl started crying. "You're pregnant now!" she wailed.

This is even worse than cooties, I thought.

For the rest of the day, I was terrified and ashamed, until that night when my parents assured me I was definitely not pregnant. They explained I couldn't possibly get pregnant from a kiss, although they didn't explain how babies were really made.

There are many naive beliefs about how a woman or girl becomes pregnant, including the fear that it can happen just by kissing a boy, swimming in a pool, or sitting on a public toilet seat. The latter urban legend appears in an episode of the TV show *House* in which a pregnant patient reports to her physician, Dr. Gregory House, that she is a virgin. "Aren't there other ways I could get pregnant, like sitting on a toilet seat?" she asks.

"Absolutely," he replies. "There would need to be a guy sitting between you and the toilet seat, but yes, absolutely."

Myths about getting pregnant are a common theme in pop culture. In an episode of the TV show *South Park*, nine-year-old Eric Cartman explains to his friend that to get a woman pregnant, a man only needs to "stick it inside her and pee." As we reach puberty, we're exposed to even more myths, such as boys promising us we can't possibly get pregnant when having sex for the first time.

The kissing incident at school made my parents realize I needed to have "the talk," but they weren't going to be the ones to do it. So they took me to a screening of the sex education video *Where Did I Come From?* I was confused by the animation, like the bed bouncing up and down, and the sperm wearing top hats and bow ties swimming toward an egg dressed as a bride. The film left me with more questions than answers. In fact, it is lampooned in the same episode of *The Simpsons* described above, in which Bart's class is shown "Fuzzy Bunny's Guide to You Know What." This video follows the adventures of Fuzzy and Fluffy Bunny as they date, get married, and then have baby bunnies. The educational video claims to present the facts of puberty and conception in a "frank and straightforward manner," although the details are buried in quaint euphemisms. In contrast, a graphic honeymoon sex scene takes place off-screen, to which the teacher, Mrs. Krabappel sneers, "She's faking it." The video ends with the message "And now that you know how it's done . . . don't do it."

Today many of us are subjected to sex education at school, sometimes known euphemistically as "health class," although these classes are inadequate. Kids tend to find out bits and pieces about "the facts of life" through friends or popular culture, while there's not much you can't find out about online. Sex education in schools should involve honest, accurate explanations about human reproduction, fertility, and sexuality, while generating candid class discussions to demystify these important topics, in order for students to have a healthy and safe sex life in the future. (Of course, some will have probably started having sex already.) In the past, the discussion was taboo in many families and communities, because sex was seen as "dirty," "naughty," or "bad." (For some, it still is.) The topic was considered private, too embarrassing to talk about, and even shameful. Girls weren't given "the talk" or taught the basic realities about sex, conception, and birth. Many women had no reproductive or sexual knowledge prior to real-life experience. Mothers often felt their daughters should learn about sex the same way they did: on their honeymoon. In a letter from the Victorian era, one mother tells her daughter on the eve of her wedding, "There are certain things your husband will require from you. It's not nice and you'll just have to put up with it"—which is terrifying advice to receive when you're about to be alone with a man for the first time. Religious views of sex traditionally taught that marriage and sexual intercourse were for procreation only. (This is still the standard teaching of some religious groups.) Women weren't thought to enjoy sex anyway. She was expected to "lie back and think of England." Having sex with her husband was her duty as a wife so she would become a mother.

I was shocked to discover that neither my mother nor mother-in-law found out about sex until their wedding nights.

Fortunately, it's rare nowadays for women to begin their married lives with no sexual knowledge. But there was (and still is) great social pressure on girls and women to avoid premarital sex. In the educational video shown in *The Simpsons*, it's emphasized that Fuzzy and Fluffy Bunny "never give in to their throbbing biological urges" before their wedding night. Most sex education still pushes abstinence as the only certain way to avoid pregnancy, although these programs are woefully ineffective. In the past, it was often thought that women didn't like having sex, but in a paradox, women were alternatively seen as whores. Girls who had sex outside of marriage were slut-shamed and labeled "loose," "ruined," or "used goods." They were told that if they didn't keep their legs closed, they might just get into trouble. Certainly, the lack of education about sex can lead to unexpected pregnancy. Women were expected to have children, but having them too young was frowned upon by society (and often still is). A girl or young woman who "falls pregnant" or "gets herself pregnant"—absolving the boy or man of responsibility and making it sound like she did it to herself—is stigmatized by the labels "teenage pregnancy" and "teen mom." Even worse was an unmarried mother whose baby was the product of an illicit love affair, her "love child" demonized as "illegitimate" or branded a "bastard."

When she was a teenager in the 1940s, my grandmother had a child outside of marriage. To avoid the stigma of being a single mother with a child "born out of wedlock," she was pressured into marrying a friend to take his last name. "She lived in shame her whole life," my mother told me. "It's sad because single motherhood and having children outside of marriage aren't seen as taboo anymore."

Madonna's 1986 pop song "Papa Don't Preach" tells the story of a young woman who confesses to her father that she is pregnant, but refuses to give up her baby for adoption. As recently as the 1980s, pregnant girls and women with no prospect of marriage might have been placed in an institution to give birth in secret, to hide the scandal of out-of-wedlock pregnancy from public view. These "fallen women" were social outcasts seen as irresponsible and immoral (while the men responsible got off scot-free). These women were "sent away" to mother and baby homes, which were often run by strict Catholic nuns who treated them like sinners. Here, they were given assumed names to protect their identities, dressed in uniforms like schoolgirls, and then forced to do hard labor, even while they were heavily pregnant. If a woman ever left the grounds for any reason, she was presented with a cheap wedding band to wear on her ring finger to give the appearance that she was a respectable married woman. If she didn't pretend to be married, she was verbally abused in the neighborhood and pelted with eggs. In these maternity group homes the women were often abused physically and emotionally. They were forced to have their babies but deemed unfit mothers. The homes doubled as orphanages, so parents, doctors, social workers, and courts coerced unmarried mothers to relinquish their newborns for adoption. Tragically, many infants born in these places did not survive the terrible conditions. In the infamous case of the Bon Secours Mother and Baby Home in Tuam, Ireland, almost one thousand children died of disease or neglect during the 1940s. Recently, their bodies were found buried in a mass, unmarked grave in the churchyard.

As a hopeful mother, I was shattered by the plight of these mothers who had their babies stolen and were never to see them again. Some of these women didn't even get the chance to have any more children.

Trumpets of the Uterus

It seems strange to us today, but in the past, many girls and even full-grown women didn't understand much about their bodies or where babies came from. But to be fair, it's taken science a long time to figure this out. Throughout history, not much was known about menstruation, and it was associated with myth and superstition. In the first century CE, the Roman author Pliny the Elder believed that menstrual blood could turn new wine sour, ruin crops, and kill bees. Others thought period blood was a powerful fluid that could cure warts, worms, hemorrhoids, and leprosy, and also ward off demons and evil spirits. Women having their periods, known as the "curse of Eve," could supposedly stop hailstorms and tornados. Some medieval Christian scholars spread the rumor that Jewish men also had periods. In the Middle Ages, it was feared that having sex with a woman who was on her period could lead to the birth of a deformed baby.

Over time, there have been many theories to explain the mysteries of conception. The ancient physicians Hippocrates and Galen taught the "two-seed" theory of sexual reproduction. They believed that both men and women ejaculated seed at the point of orgasm, the male semen and female semen mixing in the womb to form a baby. Throughout the medieval and early modern periods it was widely thought, by lay people as well as doctors, that a woman could only conceive if she had an orgasm (although not necessarily at exactly the same time as her male partner). The biological basis for this idea was that male and female sex organs were believed to be mirrors of each other, based on the man's reproductive organs; the vagina was represented as an inverted penis, while the ovaries were testes, the uterus a scrotum, and the labia a foreskin.

The philosopher Aristotle considered women "monstrous" and "deficient," because without a penis and testicles, a woman was just a "deformed male." He wrote that a woman's "menstrual discharge is semen, though in an impure condition; i.e., it lacks one constituent . . . the principle of the Soul." In his mind, "the male is by nature superior and the female inferior, the male ruler and the female subject," and women were biologically inferior to men. They "simply" functioned as a depository for sperm and a nourishing receptacle for a baby. (He also believed that women had fewer teeth than men.) Aristotle disagreed with the two-seed hypothesis and came up with the "one-seed" theory instead. This held that a man's seed mixed with a woman's menstrual blood to form an egg. This early understanding of conception was based on the knowledge of how plants grow. It was thought that the womb was like a garden; a baby was the product of a man's seed, which was planted and nurtured in the woman's "soil," much like a farmer implanting seeds to grow in the ground. For hundreds of years, this "soil and seed" theory was the accepted explanation for sexual generation.

It wasn't until the Renaissance period that some major discoveries in reproductive biology were made. Leonardo da Vinci is better known for painting the *Mona Lisa*, although he also drew a series of illustrations of conception. Da Vinci was not only an artist but a skilled anatomist, having performed dozens of dissections on human corpses and animal carcasses to sketch his findings. He is considered the first person to depict the human fetus in its correct position in the womb. He was also the first to expertly draw the uterine artery and the vascular system of the cervix and vagina. However, he made a few mistakes in his sketches. Da Vinci drew "menstrual veins" that he thought linked a woman's uterus with her breasts. In several drawings he also confused parts of the human uterus with that of a cow.

In the sixteenth century, the Italian anatomist Gabriele Falloppio was the first to accurately describe the tubes leading from the uterus to the ovaries, although at the time, he didn't understand what they did. Based on their appearance, he called them the "trumpets of the uterus"; they were later renamed "fallopian tubes" in his honor. Falloppio, also a Catholic priest, discovered the existence of the hymen in virgins. He was the first to describe the clitoris and vagina, which he also named. His findings disproved the popular notion that the penis entered the uterus during intercourse. In the seventeenth century the Dutch physician Regnier de Graaf described the ovaries and follicles, which he called "female balls," but he confused the follicles with the egg. The graafian follicle—the ripe stage of the follicle before it releases an egg—was named after him. His findings refuted the prevailing theory that women also produced sperm. However, Graaf believed in an early reproductive theory called preformation. This is the strange idea that humans develop from miniature "preformed" versions of themselves. He thought tiny babies lived in a woman's ovaries, were activated by a man's seed, and then were transported to the uterus.

More was learned about the male reproductive system when Dutch scientist Antonie van Leeuwenhoek observed sperm with the newly invented microscope. (Yes, he used his own semen.) Like Graaf, Leeuwenhoek believed in preformation. But instead of thinking that tiny humans lived in the ovaries, Leeuwenhoek speculated that they were contained in each sperm, waiting patiently to enlarge into a fully formed baby when they reached the womb. The Dutch mathematician Nicolas Malebranche became famous for his representation of a tiny human curled up inside the sperm, which he called *petit l'infant* ("the small infant"). Medieval alchemists, who were busy trying to turn base metals into gold and creating an elixir of immortality, also attempted to produce a tiny half-man known as a homunculus (meaning "little person" in Latin). The Swiss alchemist Paracelsus wrote a ritual for making a homunculus. This involved mixing sperm with horse manure in a flask and leaving it to "putrefy" for forty days, occasionally watering the concoction with human blood.

In the seventeenth century, the English physician William Harvey set out to test Aristotle's "soil and seed" theory, which claimed that the male seed united with "soil" (menstrual blood) to form an egg. He was the royal physician to King Charles I, and the monarch was an avid deer hunter who supplied him with carcasses after his hunting expeditions. Harvey searched the does' uteruses for Aristotle's eggs, but didn't find any. On the basis of his experiments, he rejected the one-seed and two-seed theories, concluding that "ex ovo omnia"—all life originates from an egg. (He went on to discover blood circulation in the body.) In the eighteenth century, the Italian priest and physiologist Lazzaro Spallanzani proved that mammals reproduce by way of male sperm fertilizing a female egg. In his many experiments, Spallanzani successfully inseminated fish, frogs, and dogs.

But it wasn't until the nineteenth century that human reproduction became more clearly understood. In 1826, the German scientist Karl Ernst von Baer, "the father of embryology," became the first person to observe a human egg within the follicle. The following year, the Swiss physiologist Albert von Kölliker discovered the function of sperm and that they originate in the testicles. He was also one of the first scientists to propose the idea that egg and sperm are transmitters of hereditary characteristics. Another big discovery occurred in 1839 when French doctor Augustin Gendrin suggested that menstruation was controlled by ovulation, which is when the ovaries release an egg. This dispelled the long-held belief that periods and fertility were influenced by the phases of the moon. The relationship between menstruation and conception grew even clearer when it became understood that a woman got her period because she hadn't conceived.

Just Relax and It Will Happen

"It'll be your turn next," promised Kate as she picked up a mini cupcake with pink frosting and popped it into her mouth. I appreciated her positivity, but she made trying to conceive sound like I was simply waiting in line for concert tickets.

We were at the baby shower. To celebrate the coming of a baby girl, the room was decorated with pink balloons, pink flowers, and packages covered in pink wrapping paper, no doubt containing pink-colored gifts. I felt uncomfortable. There are few things more awkward than being a woman who's trying to conceive having to attend a baby shower. It was rubbing salt, or in this case, baby powder, into the wound. I felt bitter, envious, sad, and yet hopeful, all at once.

Maybe it *would* be my turn next.

Many of the women in attendance were pregnant or already had children. This evidently made them experts on the subject of getting pregnant, and when they learned I was trying to conceive, they were full of well-meaning tips, legends, and old wives' tales. These included:

> *Have sex during a full moon.*
> *Have sex every day.*

Drink cough syrup.
Lie flat for thirty minutes after having sex.
Make sure you have an orgasm during sex.
Do it missionary style.
Adopt a baby and then you'll get pregnant.
Get really drunk and have sex in the back seat of your car.

(Well, that last one wasn't going to happen at a party where the only drink choices were nonalcoholic punch and pink lemonade.)

My mind boggled at the advice.

"You're thinking about it too much," said Kate. "Just relax and it will happen."

But nothing stresses a woman out more than being told to relax.

There are many superstitions surrounding trying to conceive, some of them more far-fetched than others. Many myths involve sympathetic magic—that is, the belief that like attracts like. One such legend says women trying to conceive should mingle with pregnant women so their fertility rubs off. (I tried that one at the baby shower, but it didn't work.) And it goes both ways: women trying to conceive should supposedly steer clear of "barren" women, lest their infertility rub off. Hugging a newborn baby is supposed to help a woman to get pregnant, as will accidentally stepping in a child's shadow. (But it *must* be done by accident and not deliberately.) According to folklore, many things were thought to be signs of pregnancy too. As we know, storks have long been symbols of newborns, so seeing one in the wild was said to be an omen of pregnancy. Apparently, their power is so strong that a stork can cause a woman to become pregnant just by looking at her. Dreaming of fertile animals such as fish, rabbits, or rats is supposedly a sign of pregnancy too. Finding a double yolk in an egg means you are pregnant, and so does baking a cake that sinks in the middle.

If that last one were true, I definitely would've been pregnant already, I thought.

Because these urban legends about conception still persist, I decided to look into them and even try a few.

Have sex during a full moon

Many superstitions about conception involve the moon. For hundreds of years, people have figured there was a connection between the moon and menstruation, because the average length of a woman's cycle (28 days) matches the lunar month (29.53 days). The words moon, month, and menstruation—the latter of which is often known as "monthlies," "that time of the month," or "moon days"—are all related etymologically. No less an authority than Charles Darwin thought the menstrual cycle was evidence that our ancestors lived on the seashore and needed to synchronize with the tides. According to the theory that the moon affects menstrual cycles, women should get their period during the new moon and then ovulate during the full moon, making this the perfect time to try to conceive. (Ovulation typically occurs about fourteen days before the start of the next menstrual period.) In contrast, some women use this moon theory to predict ovulation as a method of birth control. However, menstrual cycles vary in length among women (typically between twenty-four and thirty-eight days) and even vary in an individual woman, while period start dates fall randomly throughout the month, regardless of the phase of the moon. So it's just coincidental that the average menstrual cycle is about the same length as the moon cycle.

Have sex every day

Some suggest having sex every day, or even multiple times every day to get pregnant. But as we've already seen, baby-making isn't all fun and games; it can cause stress and lead to bedroom burnout. Furthermore, some research suggests that daily sex might decrease a man's sperm count. Timing is the most important thing when trying to conceive, and around ovulation is the best time, but it involves some guesswork to pinpoint exactly when that will occur. Some human mating studies suggest that during ovulation, women smell better to potential partners and even become more flirtatious, signaling their high-fertility days. (It seems many animals, like cats and dogs, can detect when a woman is on her period, thanks to their keen sense of smell.) Ovulation detection for family planning is often known as timed intercourse. There are several approaches used to predict ovulation. Many women rely on ovulation predictor kits (OPKs), which check the urine to measure the surge of luteinizing hormone (LH) that precedes the release of an egg. Some people have great success using OPKs to time sexual intercourse, but there are many drawbacks associated with over-the-counter tests. For those with irregular cycles it can be difficult to know when to begin testing. The hormone surge can be brief and therefore easy to miss, so some women may need to test twice a day (or more often). It's also possible to receive a false positive result, when having a small spike before the real one occurs, or to receive a false negative result, even though ovulation is about to occur.

OPKs can be confusing, expensive, stressful, messy, and inconvenient. (To ensure hormone levels aren't diluted in the urine, it's best to hold one's pee for about four hours before testing.) By the time the test shows a positive result, ovulation may have already occurred. Or not. Though OPKs measure the hormone surge prior to ovulation, they won't tell if you have actually ovulated. Some women experience a surge, but an egg is never released. Women have just five or six fertile days during each cycle, and eggs survive for only twelve to twenty-four hours after ovulation. If sperm is already waiting in the reproductive tract, it can pounce as soon as the egg is released. Most doctors recommend not having sex every day during the cycle, but having sex every day during the fertility window. Others suggest having sex every other day during a woman's fertile period, several days before her estimated ovulation and several days afterward. Some researchers recommend that couples trying to conceive have sex several times per week, every week, because you don't know exactly when ovulation happens.

Drink cough syrup

Some people believe that drinking cough syrup improves fertility by thinning out the cervical mucus, thereby making it easier for sperm to pass through to the uterus. Some cough syrups contain guaifenesin, an ingredient that thins and loosens mucus in the chest, sinuses, and nasal passages, so the theory goes that it must also thin mucus in the cervix. However, what makes cervical mucus watery is high levels of estrogen, which peak before ovulation. That fact aside, this old wives' tale actually *does* have some validity to it. In rare cases, doctors recommend repurposing the medication for men who have very thick semen that does not liquefy.

Speaking of cervical mucus, some women track their vaginal discharge to predict when they will ovulate. Cervical fluid that is thin, clear, and slippery, much like raw egg white, signals that ovulation is approaching. The similarity between fertile cervical fluid and egg whites has led to another myth— that using egg white as lubricant increases a woman's chances of getting pregnant, because it mimics cervical mucus which helps sperm reach the egg. In spite of the popularity of this method, there isn't any scientific data to back it up, although using egg whites is risky because undercooked eggs can carry harmful bacteria.

Some women also track their saliva to figure out the best times to have sex for conception. Saliva fertility tests check for "salivary ferning," when the saliva dries in a fern-like pattern, which can suggest that ovulation is impending. Others chart their basal body temperature (BBT) to find out when they are ovulating. This is the body's at-rest temperature, which can be measured with a thermometer upon waking up first thing in the morning. The body's temperature dips a bit before an egg is released, and then afterward it rises slightly and stays up for several days. Whichever methods are used for reading body signals of impending ovulation, they need to be tracked for several months for patterns to emerge. Many women use phone apps to help track their menstrual cycles, not only for fertility but also for contraception and to monitor other health effects.

Lie flat for thirty minutes after having sex

In a post-coitus scene in the movie *The Big Lebowski*, the character Maude lays on her back with her knees pulled in, believing this will "increase the chances of conception." Variations of this suggestion include holding your legs over your head after sex, putting your legs in the air and "bicycling" for five minutes, or the acrobatic feat of standing on your head. This advice is based in the belief that these positions will tip the pelvis and help the sperm to reach the egg. It's feared that sperm will rush back out of the female body once she stands up, because of the effects of gravity. However, sperm are chemically programmed to reach the egg and once they are ejaculated, most swimmers with any chance of fertilization will be well on their way. Sperm will swim up the reproductive tract with or without the help of gravity. If you stand up after sex, you might feel a trickle, but that's just semen. The sperm immediately head north, while the seminal fluid heads south.

Make sure you have an orgasm during sex

The idea behind this fertility tip is that when a woman has an orgasm during sex, her uterine contractions suck up the sperm, transporting them closer to the egg. The bulk of the evidence tells us there is no correlation between female orgasm and conception.

Sperm live in the reproductive tract for days, whether she has an orgasm or not. If female orgasms did affect conception, from an evolutionary perspective we would expect they would more commonly occur with penile penetration. (The reality is they only occur this way about 25 percent of the time.) For a woman's orgasm to help suck up sperm, it would need to happen immediately before or during the man's orgasm, although this is uncommon. In reality, women can achieve orgasm once or more before their partner does, or after, or not at all. The idea that a woman must orgasm to get pregnant may have its basis in the two-sperm theory that was promulgated by Hippocrates and Galen, as mentioned above. It's also tied in with the old-fashioned belief that sex *must* be for the purposes of procreation, not merely for pleasure.

Do it missionary style

Many people say that the missionary position, in which the couple lies face to face with the woman underneath the man, is the only way to conceive. The name comes from a 1920s term used by South Pacific people to describe the position promoted by Christian missionaries to replace their local "heathen" variations. (It was also once known as the "English-American position.") Some think the missionary-style position allows for deeper penetration, bringing sperm in closer proximity to the cervix. But there is no research to back up that claim. The truth is that the actual position you do it in is inconsequential, as long as there's penetration going on, and of course, ejaculation. Any position that gets semen near the cervix, or anywhere in the vaginal area, can lead to pregnancy. It doesn't matter how you do it, or where you do it either.

Adopt a baby and then you'll get pregnant

This myth also reflects the irony that sometimes, if you just relax or even give up, then it'll happen. Interestingly, everyone seems to know someone this has happened to. In fact, it happened to one of my best friends, Joe. After many years of trying to conceive, his parents finally gave up. They adopted him, and then . . . bam! They got pregnant with another son. The fact that adoption is still thought to be a solution for not being able to get pregnant might stem from the mid twentieth-century belief that infertility was a psychiatric condition for which adoption was recommended as the "cure." Doctors believed that becoming a mother relaxed the woman, took off the stress, and therefore increased her chances of conception. But in the grand scheme of things, getting pregnant after adoption is simply a lucky coincidence.

Get really drunk and have sex in the back seat of your car

This is the stereotype of the baby conceived "in the back seat of a car," and that irresponsible young people seem to get pregnant easily. (Younger people do get pregnant more easily, but there is a biological explanation for that.) It also includes the superstitious belief that if you overthink conception, it will fail, while, ironically, if you "just relax," it seems to happen magically. However, getting really drunk is a really bad idea for those trying to conceive. Binge drinking, or drinking to excess, can affect people's fertility. Drinking too much alcohol and too often can lead to irregular cycles, cutting down the chances of conceiving each month. Heavy drinking can affect a man's fertility too. Alternatively, the advice to not drink at all is unnecessarily extreme too. Having a glass of wine or two or the occasional couple of beers while trying to conceive won't be harmful, and may actually help with relaxation to cope with the stress of trying to conceive.

When you're trying to conceive, it seems like everyone has an opinion, tip, or trick, or a nugget of well-meaning advice. Many remain convinced that these things helped them to conceive, but not all of it is completely true. There are many misconceptions about conception. These fertility myths persist because they are sensational, so we're inclined to believe them over the dull and dreary facts of reproduction.

Trying Times

"Are you pregnant?" asked my mother-in-law, casting a look at my stomach.

"Not yet," I replied.

Irritatingly, people were often assuming I must be pregnant, for many reasons. Perhaps I was feeling bloated that day and wearing loose clothing, making me "look pregnant." Or if I refused an alcoholic drink at a party, it was "obviously" a telltale sign. Apparently, it was "about time" in the course of my marriage that I "should" be pregnant. In the past, discussing pregnancy was often considered impolite. It wasn't said explicitly that a woman was "pregnant," but that she was "expecting," "feeling delicate," or "in the family way." Being asked if I was pregnant reminded me of the meme that it's *never* appropriate to ask a woman if she's pregnant, even if she's in labor (it's joked about to drive the point home). This is because the question is intrusive, and what people do with their bodies is no one's business. A woman may have experienced loss, or be facing infertility, and these insensitive words will sting. Moreover, the question is also a rude comment about someone's body, appearance, and weight, and it's embarrassing and hurtful for them if it's wrong.

"Are you even trying?" she asked.

What kind of a question is that? I wondered.

"Yes," I replied. "Of course we are."

According to everyone else, you're either trying too hard or not trying hard enough.

"Then *when* are you going to make me a grandmother?"

There was the question I'd been dreading. Besides, she was already a grandmother—*seven* times over. She just hadn't been made a grandmother by her youngest son. Yet.

"It's just not going as quickly as we'd like," I admitted.

Then came a lot of the advice I'd heard at the baby shower. Matt and I had explored these tips but found them to mostly be, as shared above, urban legends. And it was awkward discussing intimate matters with my mother-in-law. All over again, I felt like I was that embarrassed eight-year-old kid, forced to watch a screening of *Where Did I Come From?*

"We're trying," I promised her.

But this was much harder than I thought it would be.

"Don't worry," she reassured me. "Getting pregnant is the most natural thing in the world."

As girls and young women, we're not taught how to get pregnant, but taught how *not* to get pregnant. In health class there may be some limited sex education, but the strong message is that we need to prevent pregnancy. It is drummed into us that the very first time we have unprotected sex, we *will* get pregnant (despite what our boyfriends tell us). But there is virtually nothing in the way of fertility education and the physiology of reproduction. We're not typically taught much about such things as ovulation, fertilization, or implantation. And when people actually do talk about fertility, they usually don't do it directly. There are numerous euphemisms for menstruation, the vagina, and the vulva, and when you can't use a word, the implication is that the body part is shameful. For the most part, we're still embarrassed when it comes to talking about sex and conception, even from a scientific angle. We blush and giggle like school kids when we talk about bodily functions. All the knowledge about sexual reproduction that we've collected painstakingly over the centuries is still often spoken about in hushed tones, if at all.

If we listened to the fearmongers, we'd think that women could get pregnant at any time. Of course, that's just not true, because most women are only fertile for about one week during their menstrual cycle. That includes the day of ovulation. If a woman ovulates, a fertile egg has been released from one of her ovaries into the fallopian tube. To become pregnant naturally, semen must be ejaculated out of the penis into her vagina, and the sperm must travel into the cervical opening, through the uterus, and up into the fallopian tubes. Then it's a race for the sperm (which are not wearing cute little top hats or bow ties) to meet and penetrate the egg. Conception occurs when a sperm cell (spermatozoon) fertilizes the egg cell (ovum). Pregnancy officially starts when a fertilized egg embeds into the lining of the uterus, which is known as implantation. From there the egg, now called a zygote, will grow into a baby (hopefully, if that's what you want).

We can get even more granular about the process. Conception is often hailed as a "miracle," and the fact that it happens at all is miraculous in the sense of being complicated and perilous. Sperm must go on a lengthy and strenuous journey to reach the egg, which is a true survival of the fittest. Each time a man ejaculates, he releases 2–5 milliliters of semen, each milliliter containing tens of millions of sperm. However, the vagina is an acidic environment that can destroy them in their tracks. Furthermore, not all sperm are viable. Poor motility (movement) or morphology (shape) may affect their quality, so only around two million sperm will reach the cervix. Of this group, one million make it as far as the uterus, but this figure is further reduced when ten thousand make it to the top of the womb. There, some five thousand swimmers will go in the right direction headed toward the egg, while one thousand sperm will reach the inside of the fallopian tube. Of these sperm, only two hundred will actually reach the egg. In the end, just one lucky sperm will penetrate the hard outer layer of the egg and fertilize it. This union of egg and sperm takes anywhere from forty-five minutes to twelve hours, but anything can go wrong at any point and there are many obstacles along the way. The sperm may arrive too early or too late to reach the egg. The timing and conditions must be absolutely perfect for pregnancy to happen. If not, the body reabsorbs the egg, and the short window of opportunity for conception during that cycle closes.

The vast numbers of sperm needed to get to the egg, if at all, remind me of the lyrics to the Monty Python song "Every Sperm Is Sacred." In many ways, the odds are stacked against conception. Statistically, a couple's chances of conceiving naturally each cycle they try are a mere 20–30 percent for women under the age of thirty-five. The chances decrease steadily as we age, to 8–15 percent for those aged thirty-five to thirty-nine, 5 percent for those aged forty to forty-two, and only 1–2 percent for women who are forty-three or over. Statistics vary, but it's not all doom and gloom. Most couples will eventually fall pregnant naturally with repeated attempts.

When you're young, and busy trying to *not* get pregnant, no one tells you that you have limited time to get pregnant. But no matter what the fearmongering tells us about getting pregnant the first time we have unprotected sex, most couples don't get pregnant in one shot. In fact, a study showed that on average, healthy couples who want to get pregnant have sex approximately seventy-eight times before they finally manage to conceive. Research shows that it usually takes couples longer to get pregnant than they thought it would. But when we start trying to conceive, we have a naïve confidence that when we decide we want to get pregnant, we will simply be able to get pregnant; that when we are finally ready, our bodies will be ready too. Just like that. We're told that getting pregnant is easy. It's the most natural thing in the world.

Most people tend to not care about how to get pregnant, until they find out that they *can't* seem to get pregnant. Only then are we motivated to understand more about our bodies, reproductive systems, and conception, to fill the gaps in information left by school and society. And there *are* some things we can try to increase our likelihood of conceiving that don't involve having intercourse during a full moon or doing a handstand after sex. (Although you can try these things if you really want to. They're not backed by science, but many people still swear by them.) Most of all, timed intercourse may help couples improve their odds. This can involve monitoring our fertility cycles by way of tracking luteinizing hormone, body temperature, and cervical mucus to predict ovulation, and then having sex around that time. According to one study, when women aged twenty to forty-four timed their intercourse to help them get pregnant, they had a 38 percent chance of conceiving in just one cycle. These chances increased with subsequent cycles, to a 68 percent chance within three cycles, an 81 percent chance within six cycles, and a whopping 92 percent chance within twelve cycles.

But this *still* doesn't work for everyone.

Matt and I had spent more months trying to conceive naturally, using timed intercourse, and even testing out some quirky urban legends, without success. Getting pregnant can be really hard.

The most natural thing in the world *isn't*.

3

THEY ARE CALLED IMPERFECT MEN

Bad Swimmers and Shooting Blanks

"Are you sure he's not shooting blanks?" bellowed my friend Sally as she competed with the loud music in the bar, although the song ended abruptly and the room fell silent just as the words were uttered. Several people lifted their heads to stare at the woman whose husband must be shooting blanks.

"I don't think so," I whispered, remembering that the surgeon had seen sperm during the reversal. "I'm starting to think that the problem is with me."

"Women are *always* blamed for infertility," Sally said with a shake of her head. "But sometimes it's the man's fault."

Then it occurred to me that Dr. Davis had seen sperm under the microscope, but they were in the vas deferens. This was *before* he retied the tubes. Of course, he didn't test again afterward. Furthermore, we'd been informed by the doctor and his nurse that it might take some time for sperm to reach the vas deferens again. As mentioned earlier, it can take anywhere from weeks to months through to a year or even longer for sperm to appear in the semen after a reversal. So, at the twelve-month post-surgery mark when this conversation took place, Matt didn't necessarily have sperm in his semen yet.

Uh oh. This was something new to worry about.

When it comes to fertility it seems there's *always* something new to worry about.

The technical term for "shooting blanks" is *azoospermia*. Worse than a low sperm count, this is a *no* sperm count, when a man's semen contains no traces of sperm. It's a rare condition that occurs in only 1 percent of men, but accounts for about 15 percent of male infertility overall. Azoospermia can be obstructive or non-obstructive in nature. If the cause is obstructive, the testicles produce sperm, but the sperm are unable to flow out of the testes because of a blockage. This is the obvious goal of a vasectomy, but it can also occur in cases of testicular cancer, sexually transmitted diseases, or varicocele, a type of varicose veins that form in the testicles. If the cause of azoospermia is nonobstructive, hormone deficiencies or genetic issues can affect sperm production. There aren't any noticeable symptoms for these conditions, other than trying to get pregnant without success. Some men also have dry orgasms in which they can reach climax but don't release semen, or release very little of it. Underlying causes of this kind of anejaculation (the complete absence of emission) can include diabetes, multiple sclerosis, or certain medications (especially those used to treat high blood pressure, enlarged prostate, or mood disorders). Another potential problem is retrograde ejaculation, when a man orgasms and the semen doesn't come out of his penis, but shoots into his bladder instead.

Fortunately, dry orgasms weren't our problem. But the obvious question was: Did Matt's semen contain any sperm? You can't tell by just looking at seminal fluid because sperm are microscopic. From head to tail, human sperm cells measure about 50 micrometers, which is about five one-hundredths of a millimeter. For comparison, a human egg is thirty times bigger and can be seen with the naked eye. So to answer that question, we had the crazy idea of breaking out our microscope to test Matt's semen for ourselves. Hey, if it was okay for Antonie van Leeuwenhoek to do it, then it was okay for us! Leeuwenhoek built his own microscopes from two thin, flat brass plates riveted together. Sandwiched between them was a small, bi-convex lens capable of magnifications ranging from 70x to over 250x. This was impressive for its day, and Leeuwenhoek's homemade microscopes were much more powerful than those of his contemporaries. Over three hundred years later, we had the added benefit of using a modern microscope with 40x–1000x magnification. Leeuwenhoek would've been amazed by the technology of modern microscopes, the most powerful of which can see things as small as a strand of DNA or even an individual atom.

Having acquired a sample for testing, Matt placed the microscope slide on the stage and fastened it with the clips.

"You seem to know what you're doing," I remarked.

"This reminds me of high school biology class, when we had to look at slides of guinea pig sperm," he revealed. "The experiment inspired me to try it at home with my own."

"That's too much information," I said with a laugh.

But we were finding out quickly that everything about fertility is too much information.

Matt looked through the eyepiece and adjusted the focus knob. I held my breath . . .

"Sperm!" he finally cried. "Look for yourself!"

I peered into the eyepiece, where I could see the sperm very clearly, squiggling around on the glass slide. They looked like tiny tadpoles with tails.

So there *was* sperm in his semen. He wasn't "shooting blanks." We were so relieved. But then why weren't we having any luck getting pregnant? Instead of a no sperm count, perhaps he had a *low* sperm count? It made me think of the scene from the movie *Idiocracy*, in which a yuppie couple waits for the "right time" to have a child, but when that time arrives, they discover they are infertile.

"We've finally decided to have kids," says the wife. "And I'm not pointing fingers, but it's not going well."

"Oh, and *this* is helping?" asks the husband.

"Well, it's not *my* sperm count!" she snaps back at him.

I remember wondering, *Is it my fault or Matt's fault?*

Am I Not a Man Like Any Other?

For most of history, you'd think men didn't experience infertility. In a prefeminist society, male infertility was unrecognized and barrenness was invariably attributed to the woman. The consequences for her alleged infertility could be harsh. As we've seen, in ancient societies husbands had the right to resort to using surrogates if the marriage didn't produce children. Other men rejected their wives entirely. Spurious Carvilius Maximus Ruga, the third-century BCE Roman teacher credited with inventing the letter "G," was also famous for being the first man to divorce his wife, who was described as "fair, good, but barren." For some elite women, having children could be a matter of life or death. After only one year of marriage, the emperor Caligula divorced his third wife, Lollia Paulina, with the excuse that she was sterile. She was sent into exile, where she was forced to commit suicide by poison. The emperor Nero also divorced his wife Octavia for supposedly being infertile and banished her to the island of Pandateria, before having her executed.

The drama of infertility was always played out in the woman's body, especially in cases where the husband held power and authority, although in some historical instances of infertility it was implied that the man was "at fault." Several male monarchs are remembered in history for their fertility struggles. Medical documents reported that Henry II of France had a "malformed penis," although his consort Catherine de Medici was blamed when they were childless for the first decade of their marriage. While fertility and the dangers of childbirth could shorten a queen's life, infertility posed an even greater risk to her rank and position. Catherine faced the constant risk that Henry might reject her and banish her to a convent. In desperation, she consulted physicians, alchemists, and astrologers. In her attempts to get pregnant, Catherine drank the urine of pregnant animals; consumed the powdered sexual organs of boars, stags, and cats; and drank potions of herbs mixed with wine. The renowned French physician Jean Fernel examined Henry and finally diagnosed his condition. The king had been born with chordee, in which his penis curved downward. He also had the congenital condition hypospadias, where the opening of his urethra was on the underside of his penis. After suggesting the couple do it "doggy style" to accommodate the anatomy of the royal penis, and also prescribing a dose of myrrh pills for Catherine, she was miraculously cured of her "infertility" and the couple went on to have ten children.

The need to beget heirs, and especially legitimate sons, was particularly crucial among royalty to secure the crown. Infertility meant the family bloodline would die out, which happened to the Spanish Hapsburg dynasty with the death of Charles II in 1700. This dilemma is explored in Shakespeare's play *Macbeth*. Throughout the tragedy, Macbeth and Lady Macbeth are haunted by infertility. Macbeth yearns for a son to carry on their name, but "he has no children" and fears his legacy will die along with him. The Three Witches predict that he will become king of Scotland, although his friend Banquo would become "the root and father of many kings," his descendants succeeding Macbeth. The weird sisters then reveal to Macbeth the "horrible sight" of a line of kings, all of whom resemble not him but Banquo. Knowing his kingship will be short, Macbeth bemoans, "Upon my head [the witches] placed a fruitless crown; / And put a barren scepter in my grip; / Thence to be wrenched with an unlineal hand; / No son of mine succeeding."

The most infamous story of royal infertility is probably the case of King Henry VIII of England. Recurrent pregnancy loss plagued his first marriage to Katherine of Aragon. The queen delivered their daughter, Mary, although Henry desired a son to secure the Tudor throne, so he determined he was "unable to have children by her"—unable to have boys: that is, the only kind of children he wanted. Henry had married Katherine, his brother's widow, as part of a political treaty. He interpreted her "infertility" as punishment from God for committing incest, blaming it on the curse of Leviticus 20:21 (KJV), "If a man shall take his brother's wife, it is an unclean thing: . . . they shall be childless." In his desperate and bloody quest to have more children, Henry went on to his notorious marital record of six wives. His first two marriages resulted in ten pregnancies, seven miscarriages, and no surviving sons. He later sired an illegitimate son by a mistress and a legitimate son by his third wife, both boys who died young, although there were no recorded pregnancies for his final three marriages. Allegations about his impotency surfaced, that he was "no good in bed with women, and that he had neither potency nor force." To prove his sexual prowess, he strutted around wearing enormous codpieces and had affairs with numerous women of the court. Although he once lamented privately to a confidant, "Am I not a man like any other?" Henry continued to blame his wives for bad pregnancy outcomes, or no pregnancy at all. Nowadays, it is speculated that he had suboptimal sperm, possibly impaired by poor nutrition, diabetes, obesity, and sexually transmitted disease.

By all accounts, Henry VIII suffered from male infertility, but no such diagnosis existed at the time. Today, we can test for male infertility.

Unsuitable Seed

"Do I hear the pitter-patter of tiny feet?" asked Dr. Davis over the phone.

"Not yet," I replied. All I could hear was the sound of my own feet shuffling in awkwardness at the question.

"Hmm," he mused. "What were the results of Matt's last semen analysis?"

Matt's *last* semen analysis? He hadn't had a semen analysis at all. It suddenly seemed like an obvious thing to do, but no one had suggested having one until now.

"He hasn't had one," I admitted.

"Then he needs to have one immediately," the doctor urged. "It's an important test that will tell us more about his sperm count, as well as how the sperm are shaped and how well they move."

The list of things it would've been nice to know earlier grew even longer. How were we expected to know these things ourselves?

"We're on it," I promised.

"Good luck!" he chirped.

By the end of the medieval era, people started recognizing that men as well as women could be infertile. (Unless they were kings, apparently.) Early physicians and scientists figured out that male infertility usually meant something was wrong with the man's semen. The cleric John of Mirfield was one of the first to suggest that men might be responsible for the failure to produce children. In a medical text, he wrote in Latin: "It should be noted that when sterility happens between married people, the males are accused by many people of having unsuitable seed." The Elizabethan physician Phillip Barrow, who published the first book on medicine in the English language, wrote that men wouldn't be capable of fathering children if they had semen that was "too hot, too cold, thinne, waterie and feeble." Nor could they get a woman pregnant if their penis was too short, "so that they cannot cast their seed into the innermost place," or if they had a "naughty or evil kind of diet." Writing of barrenness in the seventeenth century, the surgeon

John Tanner highlighted the need to consider male infertility and impotence:

> "Before you try these uncertain conclusions upon the Woman, examine the man, and see if the fault be not in him. It is known thus, if the man be unable to raise his yard, if he want Sperm, if he hath a swelling in his Stones, or if he have the Running of the Reins, he is not fit for Venus School. If the man be of an effeminate Spirit, if he hath no Beard, if he be long casting forth his Seed, and taketh little delight in the act, and the Woman in the act feeleth his Seed cold, be sure the man is unfruitfull."

Male infertility was often conceded only when the man was well known to be physically unable to have intercourse. It was common knowledge that the Spanish king Henry IV of Castile suffered sexual dysfunction when he was married to his first wife, Blanche II of Navarre. For this fact he was nicknamed "the Impotent." He blamed his inability to consummate his marriage on a witch who had cast an evil spell on him. Like the gossip about Henry VIII being "no good in bed with women," early medical practitioners often blurred male infertility and sexual performance. Male impotence refers to difficulty getting or keeping an erection that's firm enough for sexual activity, while male infertility refers to sperm quality, although the two conditions are often seen in conjunction with each other. The author of the seventeenth-century book *A Golden Practice of Physick* wrote about these so-called "Imperfect Men": "Venery may be hindered, or weak in both Sexes, if there be either no seed, or at least such as will not provoke the act. For the sharpness of the Seed, causeth the Itch . . . and stirs up nature by the spirits, in the Arteries and fils the Spungy Body of the Yard and Glans therewith, so that it is enlarged, swollen, hard, red and hot, and fit for the action."

Fathering children was important to early modern constructions of masculinity and the fulfillment of their patriarchal roles. A man was expected to marry, have children, and take up a position as head of the household. Fertility and virility were indicators of manliness. Men without children were unable to fulfill the status and duties expected of them, and so their honor, morals, and sexuality were questioned. In ballads of the period, barren women were the butt of bawdy jokes and portrayed as promiscuous, bossy, and masculine, while infertile men were mocked as effeminate and weak. The infertile or impotent man would not become a father, and might fail to sexually gratify his wife. The play *The Un-Equal Match* described how an "insufficient" husband lay by his wife "like a stone in the Wall," providing her with no sexual satisfaction. Such a man might even be cuckolded. A popular trope of the time implied that when a "barren" woman was suddenly cured of her infertility, it was the result of a dalliance with a man other than her husband. Anti-Catholic rhetoric of the era mocked the supposed "holiness" of priests and monks by suggesting that male clergy "cured" barren members of their congregation by sleeping with them. In the case of "Henry the Impotent," his second wife, Joan of Portugal, gave birth to a daughter, Juana, after seven years of marriage. However, the girl's paternity came into question given the king's widely known erectile dysfunction. These rumors were reinforced when his queen went on to have two illegitimate children by the nephew of a bishop.

There was, and still is, a lot of stigma surrounding male infertility. The topic is taboo, and men are reluctant to talk about it. Infertility has a psychological impact on men too, which is often overlooked. Men with infertility suffer feelings of failure, disappointment, and anger. It can cause anxiety and depression, and even leave some feeling suicidal. For millennia, infertility was viewed as a "woman's problem," so for men to suffer infertility was emasculating. As we know, they were labeled "Imperfect Men." To see how men with infertility or erectile dysfunction are perceived today, we need only look at the other sense of *impotence* as "pathetic, helpless, and inadequate." They are characterized as weak and womanly, and seen as "less of a man." They are ridiculed about how they "can't get it up," that they're "shooting blanks" or have "bad swimmers." The effects of male infertility on individuals and their partners can be significant. Men facing these issues need support, love, and encouragement from their partners as they manage their condition. More open discussions about male infertility, in relationships and society as a whole, are necessary to lessen the stigma that pervades these common health issues.

The Wheat and Barley Test

Dr. Davis had told us that Matt needed to have a semen analysis, but he didn't tell us where to get one. We turned to Dr. Google, who informed us that we should visit a urologist, a specialist who diagnoses and treats diseases of the urinary tract in both men and women, and also deals with anything involving male infertility. These doctors also perform vasectomies and vasectomy reversals.

We met with urologist Dr. Moore for a consultation. The walls of his office were decorated with framed degrees and certificates beside charts of the male reproductive tract. The doctor was a charismatic, sharply dressed man wearing a slick pinstripe suit. Matt felt more than a little embarrassed having to stand half-naked in front of him.

But it was about to get worse. Dr. Moore cupped Matt's scrotum and manipulated his testicles like they were Chinese Baoding balls.

"Those are some big nuts you've got there!" he said, to our surprise.

"Um . . . thanks?" replied Matt, not sure if this was a compliment or a concern.

We discussed Matt's vasectomy, his vasectomy reversal, and our troubles trying to conceive.

"He needs a semen analysis," confirmed Dr. Moore. "In fact, he should've had one six weeks after the vasectomy reversal, to test for its success."

We didn't get the memo on that one.

"How soon can we do this test?" asked Matt.

The doctor looked at his watch.

"Right now," he replied. "It's simple, quick, and it's the only test I know of that guarantees an orgasm!" Matt and I groaned at yet another doctor's male-anatomy joke.

A semen analysis, also called a seminogram, tests the quality of a man's sperm and semen for the purposes of fertility. After a vasectomy reversal, the test looks for the presence of sperm. (From our homemade test, we knew Matt had sperm in his semen, but we needed to know a lot more than that.) A semen analysis then takes a deeper look at those sperm, including how many there are, and whether they are alive or dead. The morphology, or shape, of the sperm is examined, including their heads, which contain genetic information, and their tails, which help them swim toward the egg to fertilize it. The motility, or sperm movement, is important as well, to see if they are able to swim toward the egg or if they are "lazy" or not moving at all. An analysis also checks the volume, color, and pH level, because if the semen is too thick or too thin, discolored, or too acidic, these characteristics can affect sperm health. Irregular sperm, such as a low sperm count (or oligospermia), slow sperm, or irregularly shaped sperm, like double-headed sperm, will have trouble reaching the egg and penetrating it, making conception difficult. Abnormal test results can suggest hormonal imbalances, disease, genetic issues, or infertility.

Long before the days of semen analyses, early physicians had other ways of testing whether the "fault" of infertility lay with the woman or the man. *Aristotle's Masterpiece*, that book that was read like early pornography, hinted that the man might be the "unfruitfull" one, and included a test that promised to "know the default of conception, whether it belong to the man or the woman." The couple should take two earthen pots and urinate in one each, clearly marking them for identification. A mixture of wheat and barley would be added to the pots, which were then left to stand for ten days, "and thou shalt see in the water that is in default small live worms; and if there appear no worms in either water, then they be likely to have children in process of time when God will." The presence of worms in a pot indicated infertility. This test has a long history and appears in many domestic remedy books. A different version of it was also used as a pregnancy test in ancient Egypt, in which women urinated on wheat and barley seeds, and if they sprouted quickly, this indicated pregnancy. Interestingly, there's some science behind it. Like modern "pee on a stick" pregnancy tests, the wheat and barley test worked by detecting human chorionic gonadotrophin (HCG), a hormone produced during pregnancy.

As Dr. Moore walked us to the collection room, I was reminded of an episode of the TV show *Mad About You* in which Paul Buchman has a semen analysis, because of fears that he is "making decaf," "passing bad checks," or "playing poker without any chips." He only has forty-five minutes to drop off his sample to the hospital, but everything seems to delay him, and he ends up losing the sample when his car is stolen and involved in a police pursuit. (The bomb squad later confiscates his sample as evidence.) Paul is then forced to produce a sample in the office, which proves difficult and embarrassing. The show got it right that a sample of sperm shouldn't be delivered to the laboratory later than forty-five minutes after collection, because sperm only live that long outside the body. (In a bath or hot tub, sperm can only live for a few seconds to a few minutes.) But the sitcom got it wrong that a clinic would expect a patient to provide another sample immediately. The suggested abstinence period prior to performing a semen analysis is typically two to five days. Otherwise, the sperm count will be reduced. However, waiting too long an interval between ejaculations significantly decreases sperm motility, so it's a definite balancing act.

Mad About You made the "depository room" look like a swinging bachelor pad. It was decked out with a comfortable couch, a television set, and a stash of pornography. In our reality, the collection room was a clinical space with white walls, bright fluorescent lights, minimal furniture (covered in plastic sheets), and a specimen cup sitting on the table. But yes, there *was* a stack of pornographic magazines—although providing a semen sample is far from titillating; it's an embarrassing experience. The specimen is obtained by masturbation, because other methods can compromise the quality or quantity of sperm. There is pressure to produce the specimen quickly, but not too quickly, lest he be seen as a "two-pump chump." There is also pressure to do it quietly, because there are doctors, nurses, administrative staff, and other patients hovering around.

The act must be clean, because he doesn't want to spill a single drop of that precious fluid. Then he leaves the filled specimen cup on the table and slinks out of the room, trying not to make eye contact with anyone on the way out of the office.

He Had No Child—But You

Several days later, a nurse from Dr. Moore's office called with some upsetting news. The semen analysis revealed that Matt's sperm were "suboptimal." We were scheduled for a follow-up appointment the next week to discuss his results and treatment. While we weren't entirely surprised that something was wrong, it was still a tough blow, although we were heartened by the promise of treatment for his condition.

When male infertility was finally recognized, it required medical consideration and treatment. In eighteenth-century London, physicians sold panaceas and patent medicines, which they advertised in long-winded handbills and newspaper advertisements. One product claimed to "take away the cause of Barrenness in both Men and Women," whether it had been caused by venereal disease or subsequent treatment. Medical treatises of the time understood that gonorrhea and syphilis, and their treatment (usually drinking mercury or rubbing it into the skin), could leave men and women infertile. Some remedies promised to revive the male reproductive organs, restoring the man's potency, vigor, and fertility. The "Prolifick Elixir" was for the "Numbers of Gentlemen, who, by fast living, or otherwise, had rendered themselves incapable of Procreation, have soon been enabled by it to propagate their Species; insomuch, that very many illustrious Families, who, for want of

Children, were almost inconsolable, are now blest with happy Issue, and are (under Providence) indebted to this Great Medicine for their Heirs."

During this same century, a pamphlet emerged which popularized a theory that is still around today. *Onania; or, The heinous Sin of Self-Pollution* claimed that masturbation causes mental and physical disease, including infertility. The pamphlet was named after the account of Onan in the book of Genesis (38:6–10), in which his father ordered him to marry his widowed sister-in-law and have children to keep the family line alive. Onan duly had sex with his new wife, but because the child would be considered his brother's, not his, he withdrew before climax and spilled his seed on the floor. (This act is actually *coitus interruptus*, although it is often conflated with masturbation.) God condemned Onan for this disobedience—the purpose of sex was to impregnate a woman—and Onan died prematurely. According to the author of *Onania*, "self-pollution" could cause loss of erection, premature ejaculation, and thin and waterish seed, rendering the man unable to father children. (Masturbation was also believed to cause hysteria, "imbecility," and "barrenness" in women.) The solution was a particular medicine (invented by the author of *Onania*), adopting a healthy diet, and taking cold baths, or wearing a special corset designed to prohibit the activity.

Other early sources for treating male infertility lie in almanacs and domestic remedy books, these homemade remedies known as "kitchen physic." Domestic medicine and ministering to a sick family fell within the realm of household duties expected of wives, and in many cases, the authors of remedy collections were women. Women were the caretakers of fertility, even if their bodies were not "at fault," and many recipes where male infertility was implicated worked to minimize the role of the men who were responsible for childlessness. One such cure instructed the user to anoint his "yard" with a concoction and then "deale with her; and shee shall conceaue." These remedies positioned men as the agents of cure, even if they were actually the intended recipients. One almanac recommended that male infertility was to be managed discreetly by wives with "a Confection to cause fruitfulness in Man or Woman," involving a powder that could be furtively sprinkled "upon the parties meat." These remedy books skirted around the topic of male infertility and impotence, but revealed the ways in which wives might be able to manage the male impediment without embarrassing the man.

In the seventeenth century, the English diarist Samuel Pepys wrote frequently about his childless marriage and his desires to have an heir to preserve his family name. In the very opening paragraphs of his diary, he wrote, "My wife, after the absence of her terms for seven weeks, gave me hopes of her being with child, but on the last day of the year she hath them again." He regularly charted his wife Elisabeth's periods, and wrote about her recurring vaginal abscess (now believed to be a Bartholin's cyst), which often made sexual relations difficult for the couple. Her monthly menstruation becomes a sad repeated message throughout the years, under many different names: her "menses," her "months," or simply "them" or "those." Pepys sought advice from his friends on how to cure her fertility problems and was offered many suggestions: "Do not hug my wife too hard nor too much," "drink juice of sage," and "keep stomach warm and cool." Sadly, the couple never succeeded in having kids. The modern consensus is that it was Pepys who was sterile, not his wife, and that this condition may have been caused by surgery he had at the age of twenty-five to remove a bladder stone.

In the eighteenth century, George Washington became the father of his country, but he never became the father of a child. Washington married Martha Dandridge Custis in 1759, when he was twenty-six and she was a twenty-eight-year-old widow. She had already borne four children during her previous marriage, although she never became pregnant during her forty-year marriage to Washington. Like most men of his era, the first president blamed his wife for their inability to have a child. Given her strong track record of fertility, it is now thought that he was the source of the couple's childlessness. Historians speculate that the likely cause was a tuberculosis infection that Washington contracted before his marriage. This illness probably caused a testicular blockage that gave him a kind of nonsurgical vasectomy. One of Washington's most personal sorrows was his inability to have a child, but because of this, he was elevated in American mythology to the role of father of the country. When Washington died, one of the orators at his funeral said, "Americans! He had no child—but you."

It Only Gets Worse Over Time

Dr. Moore strolled into the office with a bag of golf clubs slung over his shoulder. Gone was his snazzy suit; this time he was dressed in checkered pants and a bright red polo shirt. "I'm playing a few rounds later today," he said.

He sat down and proceeded to explain that Matt's diagnosis of "suboptimal sperm" referred to a low sperm count, as well as to poor motility and morphology. We were also surprised to discover that during the reverse vasectomy, Dr. Davis had reconnected only *one* of the two vas deferentia (known as a unilateral reversal) so this likely contributed to the lower sperm count. The semen analysis further showed that Matt had antisperm antibodies. These are antibody cells that fight against the body's own sperm because the immune system mistakenly identifies sperm as harmful invaders and attempts to destroy them. They are caused by an infection or injury to the testicles that sets off an immune response when the sperm come into contact with blood. This can happen after testicular surgery, such as a vasectomy. Women's bodies can also make antisperm antibodies if they have an allergic reaction to sperm. These antibodies kill the sperm as soon as it enters the vagina, although fortunately, this condition is rare.

Matt's issues were a direct result of the reverse vasectomy.

"A reversal is intended to restore fertility," said Dr. Moore, "but there is no guarantee it will work. Even if it does, the procedure can compromise sperm quality."

The success rate of reversals drops to a low 25 percent if the surgery is performed ten years or more after the vasectomy. In general, sperm counts and motility are much lower than pre-vasectomy levels. To make matters worse, Matt had scar tissue forming in the vas deferens, which is another common consequence of reversals. Dr. Moore took out a note pad and pen and sketched the adhesions blocking the tube.

"The sperm are using up so much energy trying to get through that tiny hole that they don't have enough gas left in the tank to make the journey to the egg," he said.

This scarring could eventually seal the tubes entirely.

We were discouraged by Matt's diagnosis of male factor infertility. Collectively, all of these problems make it *much* harder for a couple to have a baby.

Male factor infertility refers to any health issues the man has that lower the chances of his partner getting pregnant. It affects about 10 percent of the male population, and is on the rise. A recent study shows that sperm counts have declined by nearly 60 percent over the past forty years among European, North American, and Australian men. As we've seen, the causes of male infertility are many and include sperm disorders, but also genetic conditions, hormone problems, and taking certain medications. These problems can be hard to diagnose because men have no clue they have male factor infertility until they are trying to conceive. Furthermore, male infertility is overshadowed by the default suspicion of female infertility.

"The good news is that with treatment, many men who have male factor infertility can still become fathers," said Dr. Moore.

"What's the treatment?" I asked, trying to remain hopeful.

"I can redo the vasectomy reversal," he offered.

Matt shuddered at the thought of having yet another surgery on his family jewels.

"Or we can experiment with medication."

Some medications can improve sperm quality and quantity. Surprisingly, the same fertility drugs that stimulate ovulation in women also stimulate sperm production in men. For example, clomiphene citrate (Clomid) is an estrogen blocker. When men take it, it triggers the pituitary gland to make more luteinizing hormone (LH) and follicle-stimulating hormone (FSH). These are critical to women's fertility, while in men, higher levels of these hormones can improve sperm count, morphology, and motility. They also stimulate the testicles to increase levels of natural testosterone, and so does HCG, the hormone that is produced during pregnancy. Testosterone is essential for fertility, although supplemental testosterone is not recommended because it can signal to the body that there is plenty of the hormone in the system already. Ironically, this can decrease the sperm count because the brain signals the testicles to slow or even stop sperm production. The use of anabolic steroids, such as those found in some fitness and muscle-building supplements that contain synthetic versions of testosterone, can cause the testicles to shrink, leading to permanent sterility. But on the other hand, some types of steroids can reverse early scarring and inflammation in the vas deferens caused by a reversal. For this reason, a course of corticosteroids is often taken to improve sperm motility. It all gets confusing, trying to figure out if something will be of help or harm to fertility.

"We can also try to improve the quality of your semen naturally," Dr. Moore said.

When it comes to fertility, we always hear advice that's geared toward the mother-to-be, that she should maintain a healthy weight, eat nutritious foods, and take prenatal vitamins. But the well-being of the dad-to-be matters too, because the health and viability of sperm are just as important as the health of the egg. Fortunately, sperm quality isn't necessarily fixed and unchangeable, but can improve with some lifestyle changes. If he smokes or uses recreational drugs, it's time to quit. He should drink less alcohol, because moderate to heavy drinking can cause his body to make more abnormal sperm. Regular exercise is important, because this is associated with increased fertility and virility. Striving for a healthy body weight is crucial too, because obesity is linked to lower sperm counts and less fertility.

A healthy diet is also important for male fertility. A thousand years ago, the Persian physician Avicenna recommended that men eat fruits, vegetables, and nuts to improve their fertility. In that regard, not much has changed over time, but now we understand why these foods affect sperm health. Vitamins A, C, and E help the body manufacture healthier sperm cells. These antioxidants fight free radicals and protect the testicular cells, leading to higher sperm counts with better quality. Vitamins B_6, B_{12}, and in particular B_9 (or folic acid) are essential prenatal vitamins for women, and are also recommended for men who are trying to conceive. Folic acid is crucial to the creation of sperm (the process known as spermatogenesis) and reduces the number of abnormal sperm in the semen, thereby increasing the chances that they will successfully penetrate the egg. A deficiency in vitamin D has been linked to lower semen quality and hormonal imbalances. The minerals zinc, selenium, iron, magnesium, and copper play a large role in the production of sperm and protect them from damage and mutations. It is recommended that men eat foods that contain these nutrients to increase their fertility, while it is always recommended that they, as well as women, take a prenatal multivitamin when trying to get pregnant to cover any shortfalls in their diet. But there are also foods it's best to avoid. These include processed meats, trans fats, and high-fat dairy products, because they are all associated with decreased sperm counts.

In addition to vitamins and minerals, other nutrients are thought to be beneficial for male infertility. Omega-3 fatty acids, as found in salmon, walnuts, flax, and pumpkin seeds, improve blood flow to the testicles and increase semen volume. Lycopene, the carotenoid that gives tomatoes and watermelon their vibrant red color, has been found to improve the quality of subpar sperm. Although testosterone supplements are out, other supplements are in. Supplementing with the amino acid L-arginine has been shown to improve sperm count and volume, while L-carnitine helps sluggish sperm swim. Coenzyme Q10 (CoQ10), pyrroloquinoline quinone (PQQ), myo-inositol, and melatonin are more experimental fertility supplements, but all show promise for improving the quality of sperm at the mitochondrial-DNA level.

There are several old wives' tales for improving men's fertility, although let's call them old husbands' tales here. But there may be some science behind them. Some swear that wearing briefs or "tighty-whities" affects a man's sperm, and that boxers, loose-fitting underwear, or no underwear at all is better when trying to conceive; there may be some truth to that. It's a fact that heat is bad for testicles. The creation of sperm is best achieved at 93°F (34°C). Higher scrotal temperatures in men have been linked to lower sperm counts, decreased testosterone, and oxidative stress, which can contribute to sperm DNA fragmentation. This is why the testes are located outside the body, because their temperature must be lower than the core body temperature. One theory is that sperm counts are on the decline because so many men rest their laptops on their laps and carry their cell phones in their front pants pockets. Men trying to conceive should avoid hot tubs, hot baths, and visits to the sauna, while their laptops should be treated as desktops to prevent the testicles from overheating. To that end, some men choose to wear underwear containing gel packs designed to cool their genitals. Others simply chill their underpants in the freezer for a while before wearing, although Matt thought that would be challenging during a Denver winter.

Now we had a plan in place to help us improve our fertility. We were feeling optimistic, but unfortunately, all these things take months to see any improvements.

"Try these approaches first," advised Dr. Moore. "And give them a good six months to take effect."

This was time we didn't have.

"If these measures don't work," he continued, "you may need to progress to assisted reproductive technologies, like intrauterine insemination or in vitro fertilization."

Now it was my turn to shudder at the thought of IVF.

Dr. Moore stood up from his chair. He grabbed one of his golf clubs and began practicing his stance.

"But let me warn you," he added with a well-practiced swing. "It only gets worse over time."

Throughout history, infertility was considered a female problem. In many parts of the world, women are still blamed in all cases, whether accurate or not. But as we can see, men can and do suffer infertility too. The unfair focus on female infertility has also done a disservice to male infertility, letting it go unrecognized and untreated for most of history, and even today, it is stigmatized. But in truth, infertility is impartial across the sexes. As discussed in the introduction, statistically, 30 percent of infertility is female factor, 30 percent is male factor, while 40 percent is a combination of both male *and* female factor infertility. When facing fertility issues, it's not a man's problem or a woman's; it's a challenge for the couple. It's unhelpful to accuse one party of being "at fault" or "to blame" for infertility. That's just not fair. It is what it is. A couple needs to face the problem together and not point the finger at one or the other.

4

A BABY IN EVERY BOTTLE

It Worked for Me

"We need to leave," I whispered to Matt. "I'm ovulating."

We were attending a party when I started to feel ovulation cramps. These are technically known as *mittelshmerz* (German for "middle pain"), are felt during the middle of the menstrual cycle, and are caused by the release of the egg. (I was prone to having mittelschmerz, which was handy because my body was telling me when I was ovulating, but I was also prone to painful periods.) Dr. Moore had instructed us to try to conceive naturally for another six months, while Matt was taking medication to improve his sperm, so we were still doing timed intercourse. Having sex in the lead-up to and on the day of ovulation would give us a good chance at getting pregnant, so we planned to dash home for a quickie.

To my embarrassment, the host of the party, whom we'd only just met, had overheard me talking about ovulation. She dashed over to us, placing her hand on my shoulder.

"You know what helped me to get pregnant?" she asked in a whisper loud enough to attract the attention of the room.

I shook my head. I truly didn't know.

"Lydia Pinkham's herbs."

That old snake oil remedy? I thought.

I assumed she was joking and laughed, but she remained straight-faced.

"I *know* it works," she assured me, "because it worked for *me*."

When you're trying to conceive, it seems like everyone you talk to swears by a particular folk remedy. They're eager to share the fertility secret that worked for them, or worked for a cousin, colleague, friend, or friend of a friend.

The sales assistant at my local health food store agreed with the party host.

"Many of my customers have gotten pregnant using Lydia Pinkham's herbs," she enthused.

This old-fashioned nostrum has been around in various formulas since the nineteenth century, and it is still used today as a folk remedy to aid in conception. Using folk remedies to get pregnant has been popular throughout history. In recent centuries, women whipped up homemade mixtures in their own kitchens, based on recipes from medicinal botanical guides. Folk medicine was preferable to orthodox medicine, because the latter was expensive and often dangerous for women. Early physicians advocated extreme measures for women's woes; for instance, the solution for plain old period pains involved the removal of the ovaries, a risky surgery that had a staggering mortality rate of 40 percent. Gynecological conditions were minimized as women's "complaints," "problems," or "weakness." Doctors dismissively diagnosed many of their female patients with "hysteria," a vague mental disorder that described women who appeared depressed, anxious, or overly emotional. (We might recall that hysteria was often blamed on masturbation.) Hysteria was treated with hysterectomy, abstinence, or sex. It was often believed that pregnancy would cure the condition too. Hysteria continued to be classified as a mental illness until as recently as the 1980s, when it was finally removed from the *Diagnostic and Statistical Manual of Mental Disorders*.

During the nineteenth century, snake oil salesmen offered mysterious remedies to treat "female complaints," including infertility. The term *snake oil* originated from the sale of actual snake oil, produced by boiling rattlesnakes and skimming off the oil that rose to the surface, to treat joint pain such as arthritis and bursitis. Hucksters found it cheaper and easier to substitute other oils, and today "snake oil" is used to describe any worthless pseudo-medical remedy. These and other patent medicines, whose contents were kept secret and sold over the counter without regard for their effectiveness, had colorful names and even more colorful, long-winded claims. Lydia Pinkham's Vegetable Compound, as it was then known, was touted as "A Sure Cure for Prolapsus Uteri or falling of the Womb, and all Female Weaknesses, including Leucorrhea, Painful Menstruation, Inflammation, and Ulceration of the Womb, Irregularities, Floodings, etc." There was no Food and Drug Administration in those days, and the outrageous claims in advertisements were simply matters of opinion.

Many concoctions were intended to control a woman's fertility instead. Dr. F. G. Johnson's French Female Pills and Wampole's Vaginal Cones with Picric Acid were taken to treat sexually transmitted diseases, and were also used as birth control or abortifacients. The word *abortion* wasn't used in advertising in those days, so coded language was used instead. Packaging spoke of bringing "relief," "regulation," and "restoration"—that is, to bring on a period. Many cure-alls were slyly laced with morphine, cocaine, or opium, with enough alcohol to ease any ailments, at least in the short term. Some remedies contained lead, mercury, and arsenic, so they were more likely to kill than cure. Today, we know that the picric acid found in Wampole's Vaginal Cones is highly flammable and the chemical is used primarily in the manufacture of explosives. But when the alternative to pills was risky surgery, it was no wonder that many women tried them, or turned to other women for health advice, in their search for something natural.

Back in the health food store, the sales assistant handed me a bottle of Lydia Pinkham's Herbal Liquid Supplement, as it's now called.

"If you're searching for something natural, you should try it," she recommended.

The bright yellow box featured a black-and-white portrait of an older lady wearing a neck ruff and brooch, her hair drawn into a tightly coiled bun. In Victorian times, Lydia Estes Pinkham's grandmotherly face was among the most recognizable in the world. Hers was the first women's likeness used in advertising and went the nineteenth-century equivalent of viral. Newspapers frequently confused Pinkham with other famous women, including Queen Victoria, Susan B. Anthony, and the wives of various presidents.

Her image was also substituted when newspapers simply needed a stock picture of a woman for a story.

Born in 1819 in Lynn, Massachusetts, Lydia married shoemaker Isaac Pinkham, and together they had four children, so she understood fertility. She worked as a midwife, nurse, and schoolteacher. Like many women of her time, she brewed her own home remedies. She concocted a special blend of unicorn root, life root, black cohosh, pleurisy root, and fenugreek seed to ease "female complaints," although some say her husband received the recipe in exchange for a debt. She freely shared this formula with family, friends, and neighbors, but when she fell upon hard times during the economic depression of the 1870s, Pinkham began manufacturing the tonic and selling it to the public for $1 per bottle. In response to the aggressive women's surgery of the era, Lydia Pinkham's Vegetable Compound was billed as "A sure cure . . . without the knife." In the ever-increasing universe of ailments the product promised to treat, it soon acquired its famous slogan: "A baby in every bottle."

At the time, Pinkham was an advocate for women's rights and was considered a crusader for women's health. Known as the "Savior of Her Sex," she taught women how to care for their bodies, and her tonic became one of the best-known patent medicines of the nineteenth century. Part of the reason for this was the clever marketing of her image. Pinkham corresponded personally with many of her customers about their ailments (for which she prescribed even more Vegetable Compound). These letters from grateful women, claiming the herbal tonic worked for them, provided her with numerous testimonials that she used in her advertising. After her death in 1883, the Lydia E. Pinkham Medicine Company continued to present her as still alive, diligently reading and replying to her fan mail. In 1905, a muckraking journalist published a photograph of her twenty-year-old tombstone in the *Ladies' Home Journal*, shocking many women who had received answers to their queries signed by "Mrs. Pinkham."

The tonic experienced a resurgence in popularity during the 1920s, not necessarily for its reputed benefits, but for the fact that it contained 20 percent alcohol and was available during the Prohibition era. Ironically, Pinkham had been a member of the American Temperance Society, although she maintained that the controversial ingredient was necessary for its therapeutic effects and as a preservative. She later became the subject of a famous bawdy drinking song called "The Ballad of Lydia Pinkham," which includes the stanza:

> *There's a baby in every bottle,*
> *So the old quotation ran.*
> *But the Federal Trade Commission,*
> *Still insists you'll need a man.*

Convinced by the sales assistant's persuasive spiel and hoping for a little extra help, I left the health food store loaded up with fertility supplements, teas, and a bottle of Lydia Pinkham's Herbal Liquid Supplement.

Horny Goat Weed

"I hope that stuff tastes better than it smells," remarked Matt in repulsion as he caught a whiff of the muddy brown-colored tonic.

I took a swig of it.

"Ugh . . . it doesn't," I replied.

As I tasted the bitter, earthy tonic, I was transported back to Mrs. Pinkham's kitchen. The modern product no longer contains alcohol and no longer promises "a baby in every bottle." Instead, the packaging claims vaguely that the tonic offers "nutritional support for women during all stages of life," with a clear warning that it is "not intended to diagnose, treat, cure or prevent any disease." Despite this admission, many women still use it, and many other herbal remedies, when they are trying to get pregnant. I did some research into natural medicine for fertility and discovered that herbs and supplements are used by almost 90 percent of women who are trying to conceive. Why? Because they need a little help, and trusted friends and family recommend them, and also party hosts and sales assistants in health food shops. Word of mouth is a powerful form of marketing. "It worked for me" is a persuasive testimonial for many people, especially those who are desperate to get pregnant. Herbal remedies are also promoted as natural and are therefore assumed to be safe. Many people like to consider nature's options before exploring others, and herbal supplements are affordable, whereas medical interventions are still expensive and invasive (although somewhat less dangerous than they used to be). Supplements can be purchased in secret and taken in the comfort of one's home. They are readily available in health food stores, supermarkets, and online, while some herbs and spices can even be found in the kitchen or garden. They are popular among people who want to take a proactive role in their fertility, and taking herbal remedies gives them a sense of control. All of these reasons appealed to us too, and so with open minds, Matt and I started a daily regimen of herbal supplements.

In the past, reproductive health was often the domain of wise women, midwives, and other female folk healers who used herbs for fertility enhancement (and fertility control). Women also learned the medicinal properties of herbs from their mothers, sisters, aunts, and female neighbors. There are many herbs that are traditionally used for fertility. Black cohosh, an ingredient in Lydia Pinkham's proprietary blend, is believed to stimulate a woman's ovaries. The plant is indigenous to North America and *cohosh* is popularly said to mean "pregnancy" or "labor" in the Native American Algonquian language (although it probably means "rough," in reference to the appearance of the plant's roots). Blue cohosh, false unicorn root, wild yam, motherwort, and tribulus are thought to regulate the body's menstrual cycles and help with anovulation (when a woman does not ovulate). Red raspberry, red clover, and stinging nettles, which are often taken as teas, are believed to tone and nourish the uterus, and also to help with implantation. The berries and leaves of the Vitex agnus-castus tree are popularly taken to boost fertility. Ironically, the plant is better known as chasteberry, the name coming from its reputation as an anaphrodisiac (the opposite of an aphrodisiac). Monks in the Middle Ages added this "monk pepper" to their food to prevent erections and suppress their sexual desires.

There are many popular herbs for men too that aim to improve sperm count, morphology, motility, and libido. Patent medicines weren't only for women. Products such as Dr. Broughton's Invigorating Syrup were called "manhood restorers" and promised to restore his lost "vim, vigor, and vitality." Modern male supplements include maca, damiana, saw palmetto, yohimbe, and horny goat weed. The latter takes its strange name from the legend that a

Chinese goat herder noticed an unusually high amount of sexual activity from a flock that grazed on this plant. Traditional Chinese herbal medicine is also popular to enhance fertility, including dong quai (angelica) for women and panax (Chinese ginseng) for men. Ayurvedic herbs, traditional Indian medicines, are also taken to stimulate fertility, especially shatavari root for women and ashwagandha for men.

It is said that all of these herbal remedies have been used for hundreds, if not thousands, of years.

Then surely they must work, I thought as I popped a handful of pills.

Beer and Baboon Urine

"Eat pineapple if you're trying to get pregnant," advised my hair stylist, Cindy, during a visit to the beauty salon.

For those searching for more natural remedies, certain foods are popularly believed to increase fertility, like pineapple.

"I was told that IVF was my only hope," revealed Cindy as she snipped away at my hair. "But then I read about the benefits of pineapple for conception. So I ate lots of pineapple and, sure enough, I got pregnant with my little girl!" she said, pointing to the framed photo of her curly-haired daughter on the vanity.

According to online forums for those trying to conceive, the hard core of the tropical fruit is said to help with implantation of the embryo, especially after an IVF transfer. This is attributed to bromelain, an enzyme that reduces inflammation and may increase blood flow to the uterus. Given this reputation, the humble pineapple appears as a symbol of fertility on jewelry and "IVF socks."

Like athletes who wear a lucky T-shirt to win the game, women or couples having IVF sometimes wear special socks on the days of egg retrieval and embryo transfer for good luck. (And in the belief that "warm feet equal a warm uterus" that is a ready home for a growing baby.) Having said that eating pineapple is a popular remedy for implantation, it is alternatively a popular home remedy to induce labor, because it is believed that the bromelain can trigger uterine contractions. For this reason, some fear that pineapple can cause miscarriage, but this is just a myth.

There is contradictory fertility folklore about other foods too. Wild yam, black cohosh, and dong quai are believed to aid in conception, but are alternatively used to *prevent* pregnancy. Eating pomegranates is also recommended for conceiving, because the fruit is believed to increase blood flow to the uterus and improve sperm motility in men. Ironically, the pomegranate was one of the first known foods to be used for birth control. References to this go back to ancient times when the Greek physician Hippocrates prescribed pomegranate seeds as contraceptives. Indeed, modern studies with rats and guinea pigs have demonstrated that the seeds *do* have contraceptive value. Similarly, asafoetida, or "devil's dung," a root that is a staple in Indian cuisine and gives Worcestershire sauce its distinctive aroma, has been found to prohibit the implantation of embryos in female rats. On the other hand, it is believed that the spice can increase a woman's chances of pregnancy. Sifting through the conflicting advice gets pretty confusing.

Sometimes a food that is eaten just prior to conception is linked to its success. A new old wives' tale originated on an online forum when a woman reported that she became pregnant after eating McDonald's French fries. The full story was that she was undergoing

IVF and her doctor advised she eat salty foods to avoid ovarian hyperstimulation syndrome (OHSS). This legend grew into the belief that munching on fries as a post-sex snack will help with conception. According to folklore, other foods are thought to increase the odds of getting pregnant, including honey, cinnamon, onion, garlic, green tea, apples, and dark chocolate. It's also said that cold foods and drinks should be avoided, in the belief that warm foods and drinks keep the body, and therefore the uterus, warm (just like the IVF socks).

Knowing what foods are recommended by folklore to aid in conception, I wanted to know what foods are recommended by the experts. Like the foods suggested for improving men's fertility, doctors advise that women have a diverse diet including lean protein, eggs and dairy, whole grains, fruit and vegetables, beans and lentils, and nuts and seeds, all organic where possible. Doctors also recommend that women trying to conceive take a prenatal multivitamin that includes B vitamins, especially folic acid to prevent congenital disabilities, and also vitamins C, D, and E, and calcium, iron, magnesium, selenium, and zinc. They suggest that people who are trying to get pregnant avoid fast food and refined carbohydrates (like French fries!), and limit their intake of coffee and alcohol. It seemed to me that this healthy diet is good for *all* women, but in and of itself will not necessarily help a woman to get pregnant.

"You should also experiment with aphrodisiacs," Cindy added as she blow-dried my hair.

"Like what?" I asked.

"Bananas, carrots, and cucumbers . . . just eat anything that looks like a dick."

Aphrodisiacs are foods and other substances that are believed to stimulate sexual desire and enhance fertility. This belief is also a type of sympathetic magic—that some foods resemble the body parts they're good for, and especially sexual organs. For example, eating fish roe or chicken eggs is said to be good for a woman's eggs, while ginseng is thought to be good for a man's libido, because the root looks a bit like an erection. Known for their suggestive phallic shapes, bananas, carrots, and cucumbers are apparently good for male genitalia, along with nuts and avocados, because they resemble testicles. The word *avocado* comes from the Nahuatl *ahuácatl*, which translates to "testicle," inspired by the shape and size of the fruit and the way it grows in pairs. In ancient Egypt, the humble lettuce was eaten to boost sex drive, because its milky white sap resembled semen. Similarly, foods that are shaped like ovaries, including olives, oysters, cherries, and figs are associated with female fertility.

In other cultures, more exotic aphrodisiacs might require a sense of adventure and a bit of courage to try, such as cobra blood and fertilized duck eggs, which are believed to increase libido and boost fertility. In China there is a traditional saying, "Yi xing bu xing," which roughly means, "If you eat an organ of an animal, then it's good for your corresponding organ." The sea cucumber is a delicacy in China, a phallic-shaped creature that squirts a sticky liquid when threatened by predators. Across Asia, where it is taken in soup or soaked in rice, tiger penis is believed by some to be a natural Viagra. (Sadly, the illegal trade in tiger body parts is driving them to the brink of extinction.) Guo Li Zhuang, a restaurant in Beijing, once specialized in serving the penises and testicles of different species, from donkey to dog and sheep to snake, in the belief that eating male genitalia enhances virility, fertility, and sexual prowess. In

India, consuming the umbilical cord or placenta from a newborn baby is believed to promote fertility in women.

I wasn't prepared to try piranha soup, a traditional fertility remedy in Brazil, or to drink a cocktail of beer and baboon urine, a popular fertility ritual in Zimbabwe, but my research into foods for fertility was a good excuse to eat some chocolate.

Voodoo and Hoodoo

"Do you want something to drink?" I asked my friend Sarah, who was visiting from New Orleans.

"Sure," she replied. "I'll have whatever you're having."

So I brewed a pot of red raspberry leaf tea. As I poured the steaming hot drink into cups, I breathed in its fresh, grassy scent. The name suggested it would taste like delicious, sweet raspberries, but it didn't. Like a metaphor for infertility, it seemed that all remedies tasted bitter.

Sarah sipped her drink and twisted her face. "I was hoping for a glass of wine," she admitted. "What's this stuff?"

"It's red raspberry leaf tea," I replied. "It's supposed to help me get pregnant."

Sarah nodded sagely. "In that case, you need to go to Yosemite National Park," she advised. "I went there for a dirty weekend with an ex-boyfriend. I was forty years old at the time, but I got pregnant because of all the negative ions from the waterfalls," she said, waving her hands about in the air.

Sarah was a self-described "old hippie," having grown up in Berkeley, California, during the 1960s and '70s. She believed in lots of New Age-y things like crystals and participating in drum circles.

Feeling curious, I looked into negative ions and learned they are invisible, odorless, tasteless molecules that we inhale in natural environments, such as waterfalls, beaches, and mountains, or following a thunderstorm. They occur when air molecules break up due to sunlight, radiation, and moving air and water. They are believed to increase serotonin levels, helping to alleviate depression and stress. Like Sarah, some believe that exposure to high concentrations of negative ions can help a woman to fall pregnant naturally. Whether true or not, it was a good excuse to take a trip to the Rocky Mountains to test out the theory the next time I was ovulating.

"You should also try magic to help you get pregnant," suggested Sarah, her parting words as she left to return home that day. Her time spent living in the French Quarter of New Orleans had brought out her witchy side. "I'm going to send you something to help."

A week later, I received a package postmarked "New Orleans, Louisiana." It was from Sarah. Inside there were two red drawstring bags and a card that read: "These gris gris bags invoke the spirit of Marie Laveau. They help create both passion and fertility. Women carry the bag in the left pocket or purse. Men in the right pocket. You may also leave it between the mattress and box springs in the middle of the bed. May the blessings of the spirits be with you!"

Gris gris (meaning "gray gray" in French) are Voodoo talismans believed to attract money, good luck, or even a baby. Voodoo is a blend of Catholicism and traditional religions of West Africa, including magic and a belief in spirits. Marie Laveau, the Voodoo Queen of New Orleans, was a Creole practitioner of Voodoo, and also an herbalist and midwife. In the nineteenth century, people sought her wisdom on diverse matters of finances, career, love, and fertility. It's said that Laveau had fifteen children, including two sets of twins and one set of triplets, who were conceived after performing fertility rituals. For her clients with fertility troubles, Laveau made gris gris containing roots, herbs, and spices. These bags were then consecrated in a ceremony where Voodoo spirits, or "loa," were invoked to grant the request. Modern versions of these bags are filled with feathers, crystals, and other symbolic items. My gris gris bags smelled like lavender, reminding me of scented drawer sachets. By tradition, they are supposed to be worn or carried as you go about your day and focus on your desires. It's a way of carrying a prayer or a spell. The whole thing seemed like hocus-pocus to me, but it was worth a shot. I stashed one gris-gris in my purse and handed the other to Matt.

"Put this in your right pocket," I instructed him. "It's a magical Voodoo bag."

He raised an eyebrow, but duly stuffed the bag in the right pocket of his jeans.

In the days of wise women and witch-healers, magic was the science of its time. When all else fails, many modern women are still willing to try a little magic to get pregnant. I searched through books at my local library and scoured the web for any magical tips and tricks to help my chances. I learned that Voodoo dolls aren't only effigies stuck with pins to place curses on enemies, but are also used for good, in spells to help a woman conceive, or kept as talismans to attract pregnancy. Like gris gris, they might be stuffed with herbs and other mystical ingredients, or they might be fashioned from wax, clay, or branches.

Closely related to Voodoo is Hoodoo, a type of homegrown folk magic that arose in the southern United States during the days of enslavement. (Hoodoo probably comes from the Hausa word *hu'du'ba*, which meant to "produce retribution.") Marie Laveau was famous for her Hoodoo fertility potions, which contained cinnamon, sage, and rose, although more sensational accounts say she used semen and menstrual blood in her spells. As we've seen, intimate bodily fluids were often believed to have potent magical powers.

Not everyone has access to a Hoodoo priestess, so some women perform their own fertility rituals at home. Candle-burning spells are popular, which involve lighting a candle "dressed" with fragrant oils, dried flowers, and herbs, and reciting an incantation. Sarah emailed me a famous Hoodoo egg fertility spell. The ritual seemed simple, so I decided to try it. Following the instructions, I took an egg and rubbed it clockwise in a circle on my belly three times as I chanted the words, "Life of an egg, life of a child." I felt more than a little silly doing so, but I would take all the help I could get. I then buried the egg in my backyard, where I had to water it daily, to encourage an embryo to grow. A long-held medieval belief was that if a woman was "barren," a friend should give her parsley seeds to plant in the garden. As the parsley grew, a child would grow inside of her. Spells like this, which use symbols of fertility such as eggs and seeds, are another kind of sympathetic magic that follows the rule of "like effects like." The wedding tradition of throwing rice, rose petals, or confetti at the newlyweds relates to fertility. In the past, seeds, nuts, and grains were tossed over the couple to ensure a fruitful marriage. Wedding customs are replete with fertility symbolism, including the wedding cake. In ancient Rome, a marriage was sealed when the groom broke a barley cake over his bride's head to bring them good luck and fertility.

Symbols of fertile animals might be woven into fertility rituals, including fish, because they lay hundreds of eggs at a time, and also goats, pigs, snakes, spiders, and rats, which all possess great fecundity. Rabbits breed like rabbits, as the saying goes, and they start their reproductive life as early as three months of age. Does are induced ovulators, which means that ovulation is stimulated by intercourse, so they can get pregnant straight after mating at any time. Their gestation period is only one month, and a doe can become pregnant again almost immediately after giving birth. Some women carry charms of these fertile animals, with the hopes that their reproductive powers will rub off. As we've seen, the Woman of Willendorf and other Venus statues have been used around the world for tens of thousands of years to ensure that women are fruitful and men are potent. To this day, there is a strong belief in fertility charms and figurines, which are easily found online. I read of several cases in which a fertility doll had been passed down from generation to generation within a family, or shared among friends, the recipient becoming pregnant soon thereafter.

Some believe that if you rub a fertility statue, its fertility will rub off onto you. A traveling display at the Ripley's Believe It or Not! museum features two fertility statues carved out of ebony by Baoulé people from the Côte d'Ivorie. It's said that thousands of women have fallen pregnant after touching these statues, even though many had been told by doctors that they would never conceive.

These kinds of beliefs and practices exist all around the globe. At the Pasupatinâtha temple in Kathmandu, Nepal, people visit the shrine of Unmatta Bhairava, the god of fertility, where they touch the statue's large erect penis to be assured of having children. The Kanayama shrine in Kawasaki, Japan, is a holy site for infertile people, where a large steel phallus is on display for visitors to rub for fertility. The statue was erected (no pun intended!) in memory of an old Shinto legend in which a demon fell in love with a woman and hid inside her vagina. Such was its jealousy that whenever she tried to marry, it proceeded to bite off the penis of her groom on their wedding night. The woman sought the help of a blacksmith, who fashioned a phallus out of iron, which broke the demon's teeth and also broke the spell. Kanamara Matsuri is the annual Japanese Penis Festival in Kawasaki, where revelers celebrate the penis and fertility, in the face of the country's declining birth rates.

Across cultures and time, many rituals and ceremonies have been associated with infertility. In ancient Greece, a woman facing infertility was as likely to consult an oracle at a temple as a physician. Early writing on lead tablets shows that women having difficulty getting pregnant consulted the famous oracle of Zeus and Dione at Dodona in Epirus. "Will there be children for me?" they asked. In one story, Ithmonike of Pellene made a pilgrimage to the Temple of Asklepios at Epidaurus to pray for pregnancy. She was granted her wish and fell pregnant, but suffered three years of pregnancy, because she had neglected to also ask for childbirth. At the Temple of Juno Moneta in Rome, women made offerings of clothing, flowers, and fruit to Juno, the goddess of childbirth and fertility. Priests to the god Pan would also receive infertile women at the temple and flagellate their naked bodies with a goatskin whip, because goats were famed for their sexual prowess. (Just like the ones of horny goat weed fame.) Celebrated for hundreds of years, Lupercalia was a Roman pagan festival of fertility. The event began at a cave in Lupercal, where tradition holds that Romulus and Remus, the mythological founders of Rome, were suckled by a she-wolf. After feasting and drinking, priests who were dressed in the skins of sacrificed goats ran through the city, flogging the bellies of infertile women with a goatskin whip to make them fertile. The Greek philosopher Plutarch wrote about the event, saying that many women would purposely get lashed, "and like children at school present their hands to be struck, believing that the pregnant will thus be helped in delivery, and the barren to pregnancy."

Reflecting Voodoo's mix of Catholicism and spiritism, Marie Laveau used to light a candle to Erzuli, the Voodoo spirit of love and fertility, but she also prayed for the intercession of the Catholic saints of infertility, like St. Sarah, the Jewish matriarch who gave birth at the age of ninety.

"I was named after her," my friend Sarah told me. "She had a baby in her older age, just like me. If we can do it, so can you!"

From Crystals to Curses

"I've got something to help you get pregnant," said my friend Kathy. We were having coffee together when she handed me a small gift bag. All of my friends wanted to help in their own ways, sharing their personal stories, giving advice, or gifting trinkets they believed would bring me good luck. I opened the bag, and inside was a leather cord necklace threaded with silver daisies and pine cones, surrounding a heart-shaped rose quartz pendant.

"It's a fertility necklace," she explained. "I made it and cast a spell on it to help you get pregnant."

Kathy is a Wiccan who practices "white" magic, which is used for selfless and positive purposes, such as healing. This is in contrast to "black" magic, which is used for selfish or harmful purposes.

Kathy was child-free by choice. She had never wanted children, but she understood the uncontrollable urge I felt to be a mother, and she wanted to help somehow. I was deeply touched by her gesture.

"You must wear it in order for the spell to work," Kathy insisted as she clasped the necklace around my neck.

It was very heavy, and the crystal felt cold against my skin.

Crystals have been used since ancient times to help with fertility issues. In the Bible, Rachel's eventual fruitfulness is attributed to mandrakes, a plant that was believed at the time to cure sterility because the fork-shaped root resembled a woman's thighs. Rachel bargained with her sister Leah to have the plants in exchange for a night with their husband, Jacob. (The tryst resulted in Jacob and Leah's fifth son.) The mandrakes had been found by Jacob and Leah's firstborn son, Reuben (Genesis 30:14–16), who, according to rabbinic interpretation of the book of Numbers, was associated with a red gemstone. For this long-winded reason, red-colored gemstones, including ruby, garnet, and carnelian, became associated with fertility. An old Jewish folk remedy suggests women wanting children should wear ruby jewelry or drink a fertility potion made of powdered rubies mixed with red wine.

Moonstone is also believed to increase a woman's fertility, and brides traditionally wore the milky white stone in rings or pendants to ensure fruitfulness on their wedding night. Some women even wore a moonstone sewn into their underpants to ensure fertility. Emerald, green aventurine, and jade are believed to help women conceive, because green signifies growth, rebirth, and fertility. Rose quartz is also thought to increase fertility, and the pale pink stone is popularly worn on fertility bracelets or necklaces, like the one Kathy made for me.

"As you wear the necklace, you need to will it to work," she added.

Some people believe that the ability to conceive is just a state of mind—that you'll be able to get pregnant if you simply will it to happen. The "law of attraction" philosophy is that we attract into our lives whatever we focus on. It's said that you should tell the universe what you want, and the universe will manifest your goals. The self-help guru Napoleon Hill once said, "Thoughts are things . . . powerful things, when mixed with definiteness of purpose, persistence, and a burning desire for their translation into riches or other material objects." According to this theory, thoughts can be turned into things, including a baby. To achieve this, some women use positive self-talk to invite their baby-to-be into their lives. Positive affirmations such as "I am fertile," "My body is ready to create life," and "I can't wait to meet my child" are to be written down and expressed aloud, until they come true. Conversely, self-blame—"It's all my fault that I'm not getting pregnant"—and negative beliefs— "I'll *never* have a baby"—are believed to be detrimental, because the body is listening and will actualize these bad thoughts.

Kathy also suggested I create a baby altar to set my intentions to conceive: a physical space decorated with a baby photograph of each parent-to-be, baby booties, a pacifier, fertility crystals, and other objects symbolizing a child-to-be. Matt and I should also start addressing each other as "Mommy" and "Daddy" to make it come true.

Matt soon joined us at the coffee shop.

"What are you two ladies doing?" he asked.

"I'm helping your wife to get pregnant!" said Kathy with a witchy cackle.

. . .

"But be warned that infertility can also be the sign of a curse," Sarah had told me.

Infertility is often talked about as being a "curse," and it certainly feels like you're cursed when you're going through it. But some people take this literally. As we've seen, in the Scriptures fertility was a gift, while infertility was a divine curse or punishment. In the Middle Ages, infertility was viewed in a superstitious way, and the inability to get pregnant or stay pregnant was attributed to the work of malicious spirits, demons, or witches. During the European witch craze of the fourteenth to seventeenth centuries, women who were childless, unmarried, or widowed were socially stigmatized and targeted as witches. Healing "wise women" were also discredited as harmful "witches." Many were tortured in an attempt to extract a bogus "confession," and then were burned at the stake. The *Malleus Maleficarum* ("Hammer of Witches"), the fifteenth-century German treatise on witchcraft, claimed that witches caused infertility; their spells or sideways glances could poison a man's seed or render his sexual organs useless. The book says that witchcraft could freeze a man's desire for intercourse, disturb his imagination to make a woman appear loathsome, and prevent his erections. We might remember the case of King Henry IV, "the Impotent," who blamed his inability to consummate his first marriage on an evil spell.

In the past, curses that caused infertility needed to be removed with rituals or even an exorcism. This belief is still common around the world. A recent study showed that a third of Middle Eastern women believed that their infertility was a result of being given the evil eye by an enemy. One treatment for this is Ruqyah, reciting verses from the Qur'an, to drive away the *jinn* ("demons") and sorcery that caused the infertility. Muslim women might also drink holy water, fast, or make a pilgrimage to a holy site, such as Mecca, to restore their fertility. A protective amulet, which might be worn to ward off evil spirits such as an evil eye, may also be used as a talisman to attract a pregnancy. In some parts of the Middle East, which is facing decreased fertility too, women without children are ostracized because it's believed that in their envy, they will cast an evil eye on children to cause them harm. The evil eye is thought of as an arrow that comes out of the eye of the envious woman. The evil eye is also blamed for miscarriage, when a jealous woman looks at the belly of a pregnant woman, causing her to miscarry.

Driving home from work one day, I spotted a botanica and thought this would be a great place to find supplies for a baby altar. Botanicas are stores that sell religious, magical, and occult supplies. They are popular across the United States, particularly among Hispanic communities. I walked inside to discover a treasure trove of colorful candles, statues, and jars of herbs.

"Can I help you?" asked a lady wearing a red scarf tied around her head. She'd been watching with what felt to me like suspicion as I wandered aimlessly around the store.

I explained my plight, woman to woman, and she seemed sympathetic.

"I'm Maria," she said. "I own this shop. Let me show you around."

She suggested I burn incense to enhance my fertility, especially frankincense, musk, or red berries. "Red is the color of love and passion," she said.

There were candles fashioned into naked women and men, and spiritual perfumes to be used in rituals and spells.

"I recommend our Yemaya cologne," said Maria. "She is the goddess of the ocean who helps with fertility problems." I spritzed some perfume on my wrist. It had a salty sea-air scent. I chose several other items and took them to the front counter.

"Buena suerte," said Maria as she slipped a business card into my bag.

When I left the store I looked at the card. It featured an ornate Christian cross, and the mysterious phrasing reminded me of old classified advertisements for psychics.

> *God's messenger Brother Hernández.*
> *Removes curses, hexes, and bad luck. Solves impossible*
>   *problems.*
> *100% successful. Never fails!*
> *In the name of Jesus call: 1-888-541-TRUE (8783)*

In my research I had read about curses and black magic, but they seemed like things that happened in the past or in faraway places, not in Denver, Colorado. Out of curiosity, I called Brother Hernández. I explained my situation, saying he had come recommended by Maria, the owner of the botanica store.

"You are lucky you called me," he said, "because you are the victim of a curse."

I gasped in shock.

"You can't have a baby because your husband's ex-wife has placed a powerful curse on you. If you don't take action soon, her curse will prevent you from ever having children and you will never find happiness."

"What should I do?" I asked him.

"To break the curse, you must have a spiritual cleansing," Brother Hernández replied. "This gets rid of the negative energy that is surrounding you."

If I didn't have a spiritual cleansing, my misfortune would only increase.

"I will burn thirteen candles of gold day and night in my church for nine days to cleanse your negative energy."

The candles came at a cost of $100 each. But then the curse would be lifted, and I would be able to get pregnant.

Those who wrestle with infertility are often willing to do almost anything to have a child. This leaves them vulnerable to scams and confidence tricksters. Around the world, modern-day snake oil salesmen exploit couples who are struggling to conceive. In one recent case in India, a guru claimed to be the reincarnation of Shiva, a Hindu god of fertility. He was visited by a couple who were unable to conceive after six years, so he performed a fertility ritual on them. Months later, when the spell didn't appear to work, they returned to him. He now informed them that he had placed them under a curse, which would render the family childless for generations. To reverse its effects, he demanded they pay him 1.5 million rupees (US $21,000), which they did. The couple continued to pay him money to remove the "curse" until they realized they were being conned and reported him to the police. In hundreds of other cases, so-called "holy men" claim to be able to cure infertility, but their spurious treatment involves sexually exploiting their patients.

I politely declined the services of Brother Hernández.

What's the Harm?

"I've been experimenting with herbal supplements to help me get pregnant," I told my mom over the phone.

"Well, they certainly can't hurt," she replied.

But the more research I did, the more I learned that herbs and fertility don't always mix, and sometimes they certainly *can* hurt. Mandrakes, the plant made famous in Leah and Rachel's biblical story, belong to the nightshade family, and the root and leaves are extremely poisonous. Despite their fertile reputation, they are detrimental to conception. Even everyday herbs can be unsafe for women who are trying to get pregnant. Parsley, basil, sage, oregano, and thyme are often taken to boost fertility, and while culinary amounts are safe to consume when trying to conceive, concentrated medicinal amounts can stimulate menstruation. Alfalfa is commonly recommended for infertility, although it contains phytoestrogens that mimic estrogen in the body, and the plant has been linked to infertility in cattle, sheep, goats, and other animals. After sixteen years of infertility, a southern white rhinoceros at the San Diego Zoo gave birth to her first calf, when alfalfa and soy were removed from her diet. (Yes, other species suffer infertility too, often for reasons of genetics, disease, or poor nutrition, as in the case of the rhino. Typically, scientists are only concerned about infertility in animals when it affects endangered species or livestock for breeding purposes.) The popular fertility herbs red clover, dong quai, and wild yam contain phytoestrogens as well, and are contraindicated in breast, uterine, and ovarian cancers. Black cohosh, chasteberry, and other herbs taken to improve ovarian function can instead prohibit pregnancy if they are used in conjunction with fertility medications. Many herbal supplements used for unrelated conditions can also affect the chances of conception, including St. John's wort, echinacea, and gingko biloba.

Some herbs are dangerous for women when they finally *do* become pregnant. In the past, tonics such as Lydia Pinkham's Vegetable Compound contained high doses of alcohol, which led to cases of fetal alcohol syndrome. Today, common herbs taken as teas, seasonings, and medicine can cause complications in pregnancy, including premature birth, birth defects, or miscarriage. In the past, black and blue cohosh, yarrow, ashwagandha, and mugwort were all used as abortifacients (i.e., any substance that is used to terminate a pregnancy). The Nirvana song "Pennyroyal Tea" on the album *In Utero* is a reference to the popular use of the herb as an abortive aid. Pennyroyal can indeed cause abortions, but the dosage needed can also be lethal to the mother. In the 1800s, the patent medicine Chichester's English Pennyroyal Diamond Brand Pills was used to induce abortion, and a number of deaths were blamed on the pills. Many herbs are toxic and can have serious side effects, causing gastrointestinal problems, liver damage, kidney failure, or worse. "Natural" doesn't always mean "safe."

It became clear to me that taking herbal remedies was a minefield. At the least, herbs might do nothing at all for me, while at the worst, they could actually hinder my fertility. I realized I had to be careful about product claims. In the past, manufacturers could make wild claims, like the promise of "a baby in every bottle." Today's claims are much more vague: that various herbs will "boost," "enhance," or "stimulate" fertility. They promise to "balance hormones," offer "reproductive support," and "prepare the body for conception," whatever these ambiguous phrases mean. But these claims are not supported by scientific evidence. The research on these herbs for fertility is preliminary, conflicting, or nonexistent, and we treat ourselves as guinea pigs when we self-experiment. In the United States, herbal products like Lydia Pinkham's Herbal Liquid Supplement must carry the sobering disclaimer, "This statement has not been evaluated by the Food and Drug Administration. This product is not intended to diagnose, treat, cure, or prevent any disease."

In the days of patent medicines, the marketplace was unregulated, and snake oil salesmen didn't have to ensure that their product claims were truthful. But even today, herbal supplements are not regulated like food or medications. As a result, there can be problems with product quality and safety, with inconsistencies in formula from brand to brand and even batch to batch. Modern manufacturers don't have to provide evidence to the FDA to support their claims, so they can say what they like. The dictum *caveat emptor*—"Let the buyer beware"—still applies. The buyer assumes the risk when buying herbal remedies, and it's up to consumers to be skeptical of claims, do their own research, or ask a doctor or pharmacist to make an informed decision. Generally, doctors don't recommend herbal supplements for women who are trying to conceive. Newly armed with this knowledge, Matt and I stopped taking our herbal supplements.

Over the months we used them, these folk remedies didn't work for us. Nevertheless, many other people believe they've had success with them. Like the party host, the clinching argument is "I *know* it works because it worked for *me*." Unfortunately, these cases of apparent success are only anecdotes. They can take the form of personal stories told at parties. They can appeal to logical fallacies, such as the claim that something has been "used for hundreds of years" (which doesn't necessarily mean that it works). They can be reviews or recommendations, like the glowing testimonials for Lydia Pinkham's Vegetable Compound. People remember stories they hear where something worked, but forget the times that thing didn't work, because that doesn't make as good of a story. When someone says, "It worked for me," perhaps it did. But there is an old adage that correlation does not imply causation. Unrelated events can happen coincidentally. A woman can eat French fries and then fall pregnant, but the two actions might not be connected. Sometimes folk remedies seem to work, because even people with infertility will occasionally get pregnant without any treatment at all. Some people think they're infertile when they're really not. Had I become pregnant over the past six months, I might have attributed it to the supplements too.

In my search for help to get pregnant, I discovered that infertility lends itself to magical thinking, the belief that our thoughts, words, or actions will cause a desired outcome. Infertility tends to make us superstitious, and like many other people around the world who are trying to get pregnant, I turned to superstition too. I experimented with folk medicine, magic, and new age beliefs and practices. But it's too hasty to dismiss everything as quackery. Infertility is fraught with anxiety, self-doubt, and feelings of pessimism. The herbal teas, gris gris bags, and crystals can help some people to cope with the stress of trying to conceive, and the importance of this can't be underestimated when it comes to fertility. Magical thinking brings us comfort and a sense of control when we know we don't have any control over the outcome. When it seems like there's nothing else we can do, eating pineapple or wearing a fertility necklace can make us feel like we're doing *something*. These rituals can bring a sense of hope, but over time, this can turn into false hope.

False Hopes

"You're *still* not pregnant?" asked the woman in the health food store.

Her eyes immediately dropped to my stomach, to stare at my lack of a baby bump.

"Not yet."

"I was sure Lydia Pinkham's tonic would work," she sighed.

But there isn't a baby in every bottle.

She sounded disappointed, and it made me feel disappointed in myself. There is a lot of guilt, shame, and self-blame with infertility. Many women take personal responsibility for their perceived failure to get pregnant. They believe that they obviously didn't want a child badly enough, that they didn't try hard enough to get pregnant, or that they somehow don't deserve to have a baby.

"You should try this instead," she said, handing me yet another herbal product. "This one will definitely work."

Then why didn't you suggest that one in the first place? I wondered.

"No, thanks," I said, feeling discouraged. "I'm going to try something else."

I returned home to a kitchen stocked with fertility teas, herbs, and supplements. I was wearing a fertility necklace and I smelled of salty sea air. I was surrounded by incense, crystals, candles, statues, and a fertility altar with baby booties and a pacifier. For me, these were all false hopes. I'd learned there is no magic pill for infertility. But for all of the positive affirmations, the universe had another cruel joke to play on me. That afternoon I went to the bathroom, and when I wiped, I saw fresh red blood on the toilet paper. I had started my period. Another precious six months had passed by with no result. Some women look at a period as another chance to get pregnant, but for me at my supposedly "advanced" age, every period felt like a death. I sat on the toilet, my head in my hands, sobbing.

It was time for me to go to a doctor.

5

GET ME PREGNANT

The Right Age

"Can you get me pregnant?"

"Excuse me?" asked Dr. Schwarz with a raised eyebrow.

I felt my face grow hot with embarrassment at my faux pas.

"What I meant to say is that I'm having problems trying to conceive," I clarified. "Is there anything you can do to help?"

I was visiting my new gynecologist because I had been suffering from painful periods. I'd also planned to raise the issue that I still wasn't pregnant, despite Matt's latest semen analysis showing a definite improvement over the past six months. Perhaps there was something wrong with my reproductive parts too, that no supplement could fix. There is no herb on earth that will help you conceive if your reproductive parts don't work, or aren't there.

Dr. Schwarz examined the pictures of my pelvic ultrasound, which looked like an indecipherable gray blur to me.

"Given your symptoms, I'm concerned about endometriosis," he remarked. "So I'd like to schedule you for a laparoscopy. During the surgery I can also assess your fertility by doing a dye test."

I couldn't believe I was actually excited to have surgery, so I could get to the bottom of what was happening with my fertility. I cared about this more than my period pains.

"I've been trying to get pregnant for years," I admitted. "And my biological clock is ticking louder than ever."

"Don't worry," he said gently. "You still have plenty of time."

I'd always looked a little younger than I was.

"But I'm almost thirty-five years old," I reminded him.

He glanced at my medical record and looked a little crestfallen. "Oh . . . "

As we already know, there may not be proof of a biological urge, but there is definitely a biological clock. Most animals reproduce until they die, but in humans, women can survive long after ceasing reproduction. Humans have an increased life expectancy nowadays, but not an increased window of fertility. A woman's peak reproductive years are between her late teens and late twenties. By the tender age of thirty, fertility already starts to decline, dropping steadily by her mid-thirties and then plummeting by forty. By age forty-five, fertility has diminished so much that getting pregnant naturally is unlikely for most women. There is a clear biological sexism when it comes to fertility. A woman over the age of forty-five will have great difficulty getting pregnant, whereas a man of the same age or much older can still impregnate a woman (as demonstrated by many male rock stars and Hollywood celebrities). It feels so unfair. However, some people don't know that men have a biological clock too, which slows down considerably after the age of forty. At this time, men can start to experience decreased fertility, with lower sperm counts and genetic abnormalities, which can put their partners at risk for increased pregnancy complications. Men have been largely excluded from the biological clock conversation, because they continue to make sperm daily their entire lives. Still, the sense of urgency and desperation is arguably worse for a woman, because when she runs out of eggs, that's it.

Ageism is felt acutely when trying to conceive, where women are considered to be "old" as soon as they are no longer very young. This prejudice against later pregnancy is reflected in unflattering medical terminology. In clinical terms, a pregnant woman over the age of thirty-five is referred to by the hard-hitting term "advanced maternal age." *Elderly primigravida* sounds like a nasty disease, but it simply means "a woman who goes into pregnancy for the first time at the age of 35 or older." Similarly, elderly multigravida refers to a woman having her second baby or more over the age of thirty-five. When at fifty years old, Janet Jackson gave birth to a boy, her pregnancy was labeled a "geriatric pregnancy." (This classification was once used for pregnant women over the age of thirty-five, although thankfully it's somewhat outdated today.) Just like the embarrassing encounter I had with my previous gynecologist years ago, many women over the age of thirty experience aging anxiety when they are warned that their biological clock is ticking and they are running out of time to start a family.

Not only is there a biological clock for childbearing, but there is also a social clock. The social clock refers to the culturally preferred timeline for major life events, including having children, and this affects women more keenly than men too. Women are expected to have children at the "right age"—when they are young, although not *too* young, as we saw with the days of mother and child homes and forced adoptions. I remembered a friend from high school who got pregnant at the age of sixteen, to the shock and judgment of others. She left school, never to return. (But the father of her baby *did* get to stay in school.) Women have a short fertility window, but in that same window they must also go to school and have a career. It seems to be the responsible thing to do to wait until you are mature enough and financially secure before becoming a parent. But women who wait until they feel ready to be a good mother may be criticized as "picky" for trying to find a suitable partner or "selfish" for wanting to have a career. Men don't have this same conflict. Today, more women focus on their education and career first, so they are having children in their thirties, forties, and beyond. For the first time in human history, women in their thirties are having more kids than women in their twenties. Infertility is often the price to pay for waiting, although assisted reproductive technologies can extend fertility (to a degree). First-time births to older mothers are on the rise. "Forty is the new thirty," Dr. Joanne Stone said to *CBS News*. "Everybody's older. If you have somebody that's twenty-eight, it's like a teen pregnancy."

Despite this trend, some older parents experience social stigma. They may be told, rudely, that they are "too old" to have children at their age. Strangers may even assume that older parents are instead *grand*parents. But of course, this isn't as much of a problem for men, and especially those in the public eye. Most people barely batted an eye when George Clooney became a first-time father of twins at the age of fifty-five, or when Steve Martin welcomed his first child at sixty-seven. Paul McCartney had his fifth child at the age of sixty-one, while Mick Jagger had his eighth child at seventy-three. Some men get a second chance at fatherhood when they marry younger wives or get married a second time. "Second-time dads" or "starting-over dads," they're called. Both Michael Douglas and Alec Baldwin were in their fifties when they remarried and had more children with much younger women. In comparison, my mother was just thirty-one when she had me—only a few years younger than I was when I sat down in Dr. Schwarz's office, asking for help—although back then, my mother was branded an "older mom." Women are either judged for being "too young" or "too old" to have a baby. There never seems to be a "right age" for women.

I started menstruating when I was fifteen years old, which is a bit later than others—the average girl gets her first period around twelve years of age. With dismay I realized that at my age, I'd been menstruating for almost two decades. I made the grim calculation that I'd had approximately 240 periods in my lifetime, so far. Those were numerous cycles in which I could've gotten pregnant, but didn't.

I'd had so many missed conceptions . . .

If She Vomits, She Will Be Pregnant

"Could you be pregnant?" asked the pre-op nurse.

"No," I replied. The question—and my answer—made me feel sad. "That's one of the reasons I'm having surgery today."

"Well, we need to do a pregnancy test anyway. It's procedure," she said as she handed me a plastic specimen cup. "Besides, you never know when a miracle will happen!"

I went to the restroom and peed into the cup, hoping for a miracle. But it was not to be.

Years after Matt's vasectomy reversal, it was my turn to have surgery. Although unlike Matt, whom I had accompanied for his procedure, I couldn't have my spouse in the room with me. The laparoscopy was being performed in a hospital, not a Christian mission, and when I was wheeled into the operating room, it was a sterile environment without paintings or crosses on the walls. I could barely recognize Dr. Schwarz when he walked into the room wearing his surgical gown and mask and gave me a friendly wave with a scalpel in one gloved hand. Then the anesthetist introduced himself and asked whether I would prefer a general anesthetic or a shot of whiskey.

"I'll take the whiskey."

"Everyone gives that answer," he said with a laugh. "This might sting a bit," he warned as he administered the medicine into the catheter in my hand.

It did sting, but not for long.

"Count backwards from ten," he said.

"10 . . . 9 . . . 8 . . . 7 . . . "

A laparoscopy is a type of diagnostic operation that checks for problems in the stomach or reproductive system. Also known as "keyhole surgery," the procedure is minimally invasive. It involves the surgeon making a small incision into the skin below the belly button, into which is inserted a thin lighted tube called a laparoscope, which has a camera attached to it. This camera sends images to a computer screen that allows the doctor to see what's happening inside. The very first experimental laparoscopy was performed in 1901 on a live dog. (Those poor canines in the history of medicine, getting laparoscopies, artificial inseminations, and vasectomies against their will!) Laparoscopy is the most common procedure used to perform hysterectomies and tubal ligations for permanent birth control, and to remove ectopic pregnancies or mild to moderate endometriosis, which is what Dr. Schwarz suspected I had. Endometriosis is a painful disease in which tissue similar to the lining of the uterus grows on other organs, like the ovaries, the bladder, or even the lungs. This tissue bleeds, just like a period, but with nowhere for the blood to go, it can cause cysts and scars, or even fuse together the reproductive organs, causing infertility. In severe cases, people may undergo a hysterectomy (surgical removal of the uterus), with an oophorectomy (removal of the ovaries), although there is no cure for endometriosis. A laparoscopy is also useful for women having trouble getting pregnant. The procedure can be used to diagnose and treat ovarian cysts, fibroids in the uterus, and other conditions that can affect fertility. The surgery is often performed in conjunction with a dye test, one of the first diagnostic procedures recommended for women having problems conceiving. In this test a colored solution is injected into the uterus while X-rays are taken to see if the fallopian tubes are open or blocked. If either or both tubes are blocked, the chances of becoming pregnant are reduced.

The ancient Babylonians were the first to try to diagnose infertility. (But only female infertility, of course.) Cuneiform tablets dating back to 600 BCE have been discovered that mention pregnancy tests and ways to diagnose various gynecological conditions, including barrenness. Papyrus documents from ancient Egypt show that physiognomy, the dubious science of interpreting physical appearance, was used to predict whether a woman was childbearing (*ālidat*) or not. One record says, "If a woman's breasts are pointed, she can bear children. If her breasts are sunken on her chest, she cannot bear children." If her right breast was long, she couldn't conceive, although "if a woman's left breast is long, she can bear children." The eyes were a window to the womb too. If a woman had eyes "of one color, then she will give birth," but if her eyes were of two different colors (known today as "hetero-chromia"), it was believed that she would never give birth. There were also fertility tests in ancient times. A magical text written in the Egyptian Demotic script says, "You should make the woman urinate on this plant, above, again, at night. When morning comes, if you find the plant scorched, she will not conceive. If you find it green, she will conceive." The Kahun gynecological papyrus, the oldest medical text in Egypt, says that a woman whose fertility was in question should be coated with a mixture of beer and date flour. If she proceeded to vomit, it proved she was capable of getting pregnant.

Ancient Greek physicians borrowed Egyptian methods for diag-nosing infertility. In his book *On Infertile Women* the Greek physi-cian Hippocrates says, "If you want to know whether a woman will be pregnant: give to drink butter and the milk of a woman who has borne a male child, whilst she is fasting. If she vomits, she will be pregnant; if not, she will not." Also adopted from early Egyptian gynecology was the belief that women have a tube (*hodos*) that runs through their bodies from the upper mouth of the face down to the lower "mouth" of the womb. In a fertile woman, a smell could supposedly travel unobstructed through this passage, but in an infertile woman it was blocked and so pregnancy was feared to be impossible. Based on this theory, fertility examinations involved a physician inserting a smelly substance into a woman's vagina, and if the odor was later detected in her breath, the path was obviously clear and she could conceive. Hippocrates offers the following instructions: "Having washed and peeled a head of garlic, apply it to the womb, and see the next day whether she smells of it through the mouth; if she smells, she will be pregnant, if not, she will not."

When I woke up in the recovery room, feeling woozy and fuzzy, I saw Dr. Schwarz hovering over my hospital bed, waiting to share the results of the surgery.

"There was no evidence of endometriosis," he said. "But I did find lots of scar tissue, which I removed."

I was fortunate to not have endometriosis, which affects 20 percent of reproductive-age women and girls around the world.

"That's good news," I said, feeling truly relieved. "But what about my fertility?"

"I did some testing," he said. "Rest for now and we'll talk more at your post-op in two weeks."

He left, and I fell asleep again.

A few days later, when I menstruated, I was shocked to see that my period blood was blue. I discovered that having a "blue period" is normal after a dye test, when the inky-colored contrast material is flushed out of the uterus by the period.

Just Adopt

"How did your surgery go?" asked my friend Joe, over lattes at our favorite coffee shop.

"It went well," I said with a wince as I sat down. I was still recovering.

"I'm worried about you," he said. "You're going through so much pain and heartache over this."

"It'll be worth it, when I finally get pregnant," I said hopefully.

He took a sip of his latte thoughtfully. "You know, there are already so many children who need a place to call home," he said. "Why don't you just adopt?"

Joe, if you'll remember, was the friend who'd previously advised, "Adopt, and then you'll get pregnant," because it had happened to his parents after they adopted him.

Opening one's home and heart to a child who is already alive is an undeniably compelling option. In the United States alone, there are about one hundred thousand children waiting to be adopted into a loving family, many of which are older or are living with disabilities. Because of this, people who want to have kids biologically instead of adopting, and especially infertile couples who are having difficulty doing so, are sometimes seen as selfish. But being told to "just adopt" is dismissive of the dream to have a biological child, who may be born with her father's eyes or his mother's smile. Letting go of that dream can be incredibly difficult, and something no one should *have* to do. Adoption allows people to parent and to not remain childless, but it doesn't cure infertility. It doesn't cure the yearning to reproduce, the wish to have a child who is genetically linked, or the sadness that a normal and natural function of the body doesn't work the way it should.

Besides, the decision to "just adopt" is not always the easy answer for infertility that some people think it is. In the animated movie *Despicable Me*, the super-villain Gru adopts sisters Margo, Edith, and Agnes from a local orphanage to help execute his evil plan to steal the moon. Hollywood makes adoption seem simple. But effective family planning has meant that there are fewer children available for adoption than in the past. What's more, very few people voluntarily "give up" their children for adoption, even with unintended pregnancies, so adoption is not the simple and straight-forward solution it may have once seemed to be. It is also much harder to adopt today because of the injustices of past practices, as we have seen, in which unmarried mothers were coerced to surrender their babies for adoption. People can still adopt, but the system is *much* more heavily regulated (rightly so, in many ways). Many couples are not deemed suitable to adopt for reasons of age, health, or marital status. (In the US, same-sex adoption has only been legal since 2017, while as a single man, Gru would likely have never been able to adopt those three little girls.) The exorbitant costs of adoption (equaling or exceeding the cost of IVF) are preclusive for many people, because the complicated bureaucratic and lengthy process involves agencies, attorneys, social workers, doctors, coun-selors, and more. In many cases, the adoption falls through for one reason or another, causing heartbreak for would-be parents.

But there are other factors that further complicate the simplistic "just adopt" narrative—in particular, the difficulties faced by adoptees. It's often thought that children are "lucky" to be adopted and that adoption is a "gift", but people don't understand that adopted children may live with the trauma of being separated from their birth parents. Many adoptees wrestle with the psycho-logical effects of adoption, including issues of identity and belonging (especially in transracial adoptions), and experience a deep sense of loss, rejection, shame, guilt, and grief. Many biological parents, especially birth mothers, who lose their children to adoption also report feelings of depression, anxiety, and grief. The decision to adopt is not one to be made lightly, and adoption simply isn't always an option for those hoping to build a family.

Like the flippant "Just adopt" comment, many microaggressions are heard by couples who confide in others that they are having difficulty getting pregnant. Another common (and cold) response to expressions of infertility is that "the world is overpopulated anyway." After all, the command to "be fruitful and multiply" was made when the population of the world consisted of only two people. Contrary to the historical concerns of underpopulation are modern-day concerns of overpopulation and its effects on environmental issues such as global warming. Fears for our planet are valid, but as mentioned much earlier in this book, rather than facing global overpopulation, we are actually in the midst of a "baby bust" in which birth rates are declining, especially across the Western world. In the United States, the birth rate has hit a record low in which people are having fewer children than the 2.1 average needed to maintain a steady population. Decades ago, the birth rate plummeted when women were able to control their own reproductive destinies through the use of birth control (without having to resort to dangerous snake oils). Today, people want fewer children. Others are finding that even if they want a child, or they want more children, rising rates of infertility are making that a lot harder.

About 15 percent of people never have children, whether by circumstance or by choice. It is often assumed that those without children must be *unable* to have children, rather than that they don't want to have them. But there is a difference between being involuntarily as opposed to voluntarily childless. Growing numbers of people self-identify as childless by choice, or as "child-*free*" to avoid the stigma of "child*less*." The popularity of voluntary child-lessness rose steeply from the 1970s on and is linked to a decline in marriage. Times are changing, and not having children is becoming normalized, although some still judge child-free people, and especially women. They may be seen as unusual or deviant, and may be stigmatized by others. Studies show that these women are viewed more negatively than those who have children, or those who are at least planning to have them. Child-free women form a marginalized community. They are often ignored and their voices drowned out, because their lives differ from social norms and expectations. Due to the stereotype of the "selfish single" person, people who do not want kids may be shamed and accused of being selfish and self-absorbed.

Child-free people may be told dismissively, "You'll change your mind one day." Many believe that having children is necessary for some kind of "completeness" and that nonparents are somehow "missing out." It is thought they will lead lonely, unfulfilled lives, feeling "regret" for the babies they never had. However, not everyone gets baby fever. Not everybody is a "kid person," and parenthood is not for all. Just like people who decide to have kids, most people who choose a child-free life are confident in their decision. This doesn't mean they don't have a parental impulse, but they are instead content with their friends and family, being the "cool" aunt or uncle around their nieces and nephews, and having their four-legged "babies" or "furbabies." There are many child-free role models, including Oprah Winfrey. The TV host once said that she saw "the depth of responsibility and sacrifice that is actually required to be a mother" and chose not to have kids. "I have not had one regret about that," Winfrey added. She founded the Oprah

Winfrey Leadership Academy for Girls in South Africa, adding, "Those girls fill that maternal fold that I perhaps would have had. In fact, they overfill. I'm overflowed with maternal."

Then there are the clichéd comments that people with infertility hear from those who are fortunate enough to already be parents.

"You're lucky you don't have children."

"You should babysit my kids for a day. That'll change your mind about wanting children!"

"If infertility is stressing you out, just wait until you have kids!"

And the inspired idea that we should instead "buy a dog and travel the world!"

These trite sentiments emphasize the perceived "problems" associated with raising children, such as the high costs of clothing, health care, and education. They argue that children are a lot of work and represent a loss of freedom, making it harder to travel, build a career, have a social life, or find time for adult interests. We're told we'll be vomited on, peed and pooped on, screamed at, and hit. There'll be no sleep, no sex, and no time until the kids turn eighteen and move away from home. These remarks come from parents trying to educate nonparents about the trade-offs that come with parenthood; however, couples with infertility are aware of the realities of having children, and would joyfully bear these so-called sacrifices in exchange for a longed-for child. Ultimately, most parents know that it is worth it.

While these comments are often intended to make others feel better about not having children, they tend to minimize the pain of infertility. Not having children is not what we consider "lucky." Similarly, pregnant women will say, "You're lucky you're not pregnant," complaining of morning sickness, weight gain, incontinence, and other pregnancy woes. But of course, women with infertility would happily suffer these temporary troubles to be pregnant.

"It could be worse," I was also told. "You could have cancer."

I heard all of these platitudes from friends, family, colleagues, and acquaintances. When you face infertility, you can be sure that everyone you know, and even those you don't, will give you their unsolicited opinion and advice—although they're not the ones experiencing infertility, for the most part, so they don't know what it's like. Infertility is often little understood by those who don't experience it, and for them, the pain is difficult to imagine. The truth is that no one really knows what to say. But we shouldn't have to justify our personal choices to have children, or not have children. Just like the arguments about the elusive "right age" to have kids, women are in a no-win situation when it comes to both fertility and infertility. They are seen as selfish for wanting kids, or for not wanting kids. They are told they are making sacrifices if they have kids, or if they don't have kids. And they are warned that they will regret having kids, or not having kids. Why can't we just let people make their own choices about how to build their family (or not) without judgment, and then respect their decisions?

As they say, to each their own.

The Wandering Womb

Matt and I sat nervously in Dr. Schwarz's office, waiting to have my postoperative appointment. We had already waited for him for over an hour. He was a gynecologist and also an obstetrician, so just to rub it in, we'd been forced to spend that entire time staring at his walls, which were decorated with prenatal posters and charts of fetal development.

"Sorry I'm late," he apologized when he rushed into the room. "I had an emergency C-section this morning, but it all went well, I'm pleased to say."

There were constant reminders of other people's fertility everywhere.

"You look pretty good for someone who's just had a C-section," joked Matt.

We all laughed, and it eased the tension I felt. Yes, there were reminders of other people's fertility everywhere, but sometimes we had to make light of the situation to keep our sanity.

I was desperate to learn about my fertility.

"What did you find out during my surgery?" I asked the doctor.

"You have a condition called dysmenorrhea," he replied. Seeing the look of concern on my face, he added, "Which is just a fancy way of saying menstrual cramps."

It's very common to experience menstrual cramps before or during a period, and to have *mittelschmerz* at ovulation time. Around 80 percent of women experience period pain at some stage of their lives, while up to 20 percent suffer painful periods, or dysmenorrhea.

"What's it caused by?" I asked.

"There are two different types of dysmenorrhea," he explained. "Primary dysmenorrhea is caused by prostaglandins. These are the hormones released by the body when the lining is sloughing off during a menstrual period, which also trigger the uterus to contract during childbirth. Secondary dysmenorrhea is often caused by endometriosis, but in your case, it's because of scar tissue. You probably developed this scar tissue from a previous infection."

Dr. Schwarz had also removed a fibroid from my uterus. This is a procedure known as a myomectomy. Fibroids are tumors made up of the muscle and fibrous connective tissue from the wall of the uterus. These kinds of tumors are usually noncancerous, although they can cause heavy menstrual bleeding and pelvic pain, particularly if they are large. Fibroids can range from the size of a pea to (rarely) the size of a watermelon, sometimes growing from a stalk attached to the uterus. It is estimated that up to 80 percent of women will develop fibroids in their lifetime. I had only one small fibroid, while some women have dozens of them. Often there are no symptoms, so some doctors opt for observation instead of removal. But one uncommon type, submucosal fibroids, can cause infertility or repeated pregnancy loss because they grow in the open space inside the uterus, where they might prevent implantation of an embryo.

Over the centuries, we have moved away from mysticism to medicine to explain infertility. The ancient Greeks were the first to seek medical causes for infertility. Hippocrates came up with the concept of the "wandering womb." This was the idea that the uterus could float about a woman's body, bumping into other organs and causing health problems, including infertility. As the physician Aretaeus of Cappadocia wrote, the uterus "moves of itself hither and thither in the flanks." The wandering womb theory was based in humorism, an early system of medicine. Doctors believed that the four humors—blood, yellow bile, black bile, and phlegm—needed to be balanced in the body to maintain health. It was thought that if the womb became too dry, because of a lack of blood or semen, it wandered the body in search of moisture. Infertility was also understood to be caused by a womb that was too dry, too wet, the wrong size, misaligned, or misshapen. Miscarriage occurred when a woman's womb was apparently "too cold" for seed to grow or too wet for the conception to stick. These theories were still around by the Middle Ages. The twelfth-century women's health compendium *The Trotula* says that infertility is the result of a woman's womb being too hot or humid: "the great humidity which is in the mother suffocates the sperm which she receives. . . . [If] it is very hot when the mother receives the seed she burns it and therefore she cannot conceive." To figure out the temperament of a woman's womb, she was instructed to soak a cloth attached to a string with "pennyroyal, laurel or another hot oil" and insert it into her vagina, tying the string around her leg and going to sleep. If in the morning the cloth had come out, her body was "hot"; if it had not, her body was "cold," the theory being that things which are too similar repel one another.

Early doctors also had a habit of body policing. A woman's physique might be to blame for infertility, if she were too large. "Fat suffocates the seed of man," wrote Arnaud de Villeneuve. *The Trotula* suggested sweating out the fat with steam baths or hot sand. On the other hand, a slim woman without a big bust, belly, and bottom might also be barren because she was "too thin, a foolish and uncomely shape," according to Philip Barrow, mentioned in chapter 3, who wrote the first medical book in English. *The Trotula* further suggested that infertility could be caused by a "suffocation of the uterus" or a "choked womb." This theory was also rooted in ancient Greek medicine. The Hippocratic texts talk about "menstrual retention," in which it was thought that period blood could accumulate in the body, leading to fertility problems. (For this condition, the expulsive value of a sneeze could be beneficial.) Hippocrates further promulgated the belief that women could only lead healthy lives by being pregnant, teaching that women who never had children were "weakened" for life. Those who never conceived were thought to have thousands of "spoiled seeds" clogging their wombs and rising up into their heart, lungs, and throat.

Medieval doctors also believed in a kind of biological clock. As the French physician Lazarus Riverius noted, for women, "elderly years cause a Total dispaire of Conception." In line with the two-seed theory that women produced sperm too, one author wrote of "old" women that "the seed of the aged is in too small a quantity and too cold." Philip Barrow thought that an older woman's womb was "too foul, filthy and dry" for conception to happen. By the eighteenth century, when the theory that women produced eggs from ovaries gained ground, it was soon inferred that age affected the appearance of the ovaries and the quality of eggs. Scottish physician John Maubray wrote of the ovaries, "In old Women they appear dry; small, and wrinkled, scarcely weighing half a Drachm." By the mid-century, the English physician John Burton concurred, "As Old Age advances, they wither and shrivel up." French professor of medicine Jean Astruc connected the state of the ovaries to the termination of periods: "In old Women or those who are past forty five or fifty the *Menstrua* are deficient, the *Ovaria* are too rigid, dense and wrinkled; consequently they are incapable of Fecundation." Doctors started to link barrenness to the "stoppage of the terms," although the word *menopause* was not coined until the nineteenth century. (The term *period* in reference to menstruation also dates to the nineteenth century and means "an interval of time" or "a repeated cycle of events.") In the past, there was a kind of social clock too, as shown by popular ballads, poems, and jokes that mocked an older woman's continued desire for sex, marriage, and children.

In a Victorian take on the wandering womb, some physicians believed in the idea of a falling uterus. This was the concern that vigorous exercise, such as engaging in sports, could cause the uterus to fall out of place or even burst. In 1898, a doctor in Berlin wrote in the *German Journal of Physical Education*, "Violent movements of the body can cause a shift in the position and a loosening of the uterus as well as prolapse and bleeding, with resulting sterility, thus defeating a woman's true purpose in life, i.e., the bringing forth of strong children." The belief that women are delicate, fragile creatures who shouldn't exercise for fear of damaging their wombs has endured into modern times. Katherine Switzer, the first woman to officially run the Boston Marathon in 1967, recalls in her memoir how a doctor told her that doing something that arduous would make her uterus fall out. A falling uterus is not to be confused with uterine prolapse, which is a real medical condition, although it's not caused by exercising. This happens when the uterus sags into the vagina, because pregnancy or childbirth has weakened the muscles and tissues in the pelvic floor so it can no longer support its own weight.

Also during the Victorian era, Harvard medical doctor Edward Clarke claimed that educating young women would lead to infertility by inhibiting the development of the reproductive system. It was further speculated that infertility had an underlying psychological cause, such as melancholy or apprehension. The psychiatric community looked for evidence of their patients' unconscious desires to avoid parenthood. It was thought that infertile men and women might be ambivalent or fearful about becoming parents, or "subconsciously" might not really want children anyway. These theories were shot down when it became understood that infertile women were no more conflicted about motherhood than were fertile women. But it would soon become apparent that infertility was always physiological. When medical technology improved in the early twentieth century, doctors were able to better diagnose and recognize the physical causes of infertility, including ovulation problems and tubal blockages.

Down the Tubes

Just when I laughed to myself that it took surgery for me to be diagnosed with garden-variety menstrual cramps, I found out that there was more to the story.

"I think I discovered the causes of your subfertility," Dr. Schwarz said. "One of your ovaries is very small. It was difficult to see, but I finally found it hiding behind your bladder."

The ovaries are located in the lower abdomen, one on each side of the uterus, but they can sometimes hide behind the uterus or loops of bowel. Some women are born with small ovaries, only one ovary, or no ovaries at all. There are many reasons for this, from genetic conditions to the effects of infections such as the mumps, or even eating disorders. In my case, I was just born that way. The ovaries change in size throughout life too. At birth they are very small, and then they increase in size during puberty. They become enlarged during ovulation, menstruation, and pregnancy, when they produce extra estrogen and progesterone. The ovaries can also increase in size because of medical conditions such as polycystic ovarian syndrome (PCOS), or when women undergo fertility treatments. But sadly, there is some truth to the unflattering observations of history that older ovaries "wither and shrivel up," because yes, they do indeed shrink after menopause because they stop making estrogen and progesterone. (Although they continue producing testosterone for up to 20 years.) When it comes to getting pregnant, size matters, and smaller ovaries mean that a woman's egg reserve is lower than average.

"You specifically said *causes*?" I asked nervously.

"Yes," said Dr. Schwarz. "The HSG revealed that you only have one open fallopian tube."

The HSG (hysterosalpingogram) is also known as a dye test or tubal flushing. (I was starting to learn that infertility involves so many rambling technical terms that they're usually reduced to an alphabet soup of abbreviations, for the ease of doctors and patients.) The procedure has been used since it was first introduced in 1910. The point of the test is to check to see if the fallopian tubes are clear or if they are blocked. If the tubes are blocked, this affects fertility, because the passage for sperm to get to eggs, and the path for the fertilized egg to reach the uterus, is obstructed, making natural pregnancy impossible (which is curiously reminiscent of the ancient Egyptian belief that some sort of blocked "tube" can prevent pregnancy). As with ovaries, some women are born with only one tube, or no tubes at all. Other women might lose a tube because of ovarian cancer, pelvic infection, or an ectopic pregnancy. The latter is a dangerous condition in which a fertilized egg implants and grows outside of the uterus, usually in a fallopian tube, which is often removed as a matter of life or death.

An amazing fact is that fallopian tubes are mobile parts of the reproductive tract. When a tube isn't there or is broken, the other ovary can actually move its finger-like appendages over to the opposite ovary and pick up an available egg. In most cases, the fallopian tubes become blocked because of mucus plugs, scarring, or infection, such as that caused by pelvic inflammatory disease. Damaged or blocked fallopian tubes are extremely common and are the cause of about 35 percent of female infertility. The encouraging news is that the dye test itself frequently removes debris from the fallopian tubes, which improves the chances of conception. A similar procedure known as tubal cannulation involves inserting a catheter into the delicate tubes in order to unblock them. Studies and anecdotal evidence show that many women get pregnant naturally after having these procedures.

"But can we get pregnant now?" Matt asked.

"Yes," replied Dr. Schwarz.

We breathed a sigh of relief.

"Although it may take you twice as long."

During a menstrual period, both ovaries grow follicles that could become mature eggs. Around day 7, one becomes the dominant follicle, so the others stop growing. Each cycle, only one ovary develops a mature egg from the follicle, unless the woman is having fertility treatment, in which case multiple follicles and eggs may grow. (Typically, the presence of multiple eggs could mean the release of both at ovulation, resulting in the possibility of twins, if both become fertilized.) The ovaries take turns at ovulation. But which ovary develops the winning egg isn't simply a matter of left-right-left-right alteration, nor is it purely random. Studies show that, likely due to anatomical differences between the sides of the reproductive system, the right ovary is significantly more likely to be the one to ovulate. But in my case, the right side was suboptimal, with a very small ovary and a blocked fallopian tube.

We were reeling from the shock of the diagnosis. We were thrilled at being told it was still possible for us to get pregnant, but we faced some serious obstacles. We were working at half capacity, with only one working testicle and vas deferens, and one working ovary and fallopian tube. The old theories of the vagina being an inverted penis were wrong, although male and female sex organs are homologous, meaning that they have similar origins and their functions are very similar. I realized that ironically, Matt and I had the *same* cause of infertility. Getting pregnant was going to take even more time, but this was time we didn't have, not only because of "advancing age"—in terms of fertility, anyway—but also because of the blockages we were both experiencing in our respective tubes. Just like the obstructions that can form in a man's vas deferens after a vasectomy reversal, following a tubal flushing, many women eventually experience a reblocking of their tubes. If that wasn't enough to worry about, surgery itself can also cause the formation of scar tissue.

"You should try to conceive naturally over the next six months," said Dr. Schwarz. Again, we were being advised to wait and see. "But if you don't succeed in that time frame, I suggest you visit a reproductive endocrinologist to investigate your fertility further."

We left the doctor's office in a daze. Stepping outside into the bright sunlight, I overheard another patient talking on her phone. She was calling her husband with good news.

"Honey, I'm pregnant!" she announced. She began crying tears of joy.

I felt tears welling up in my eyes too, but they were tears of bitterness at the hand I'd been dealt in life. It just wasn't fair that some people seemed to get pregnant so easily, while it's so difficult for others.

6

A ROCKY PLACE

Are You Barren?

"These are for your kids," said the bank teller as he handed me a couple of rainbow-colored lollipops.

"Thanks, but I don't have any," I replied.

He looked at me like I had horns growing out of my head.

"Why not?" he asked.

Over the years, the question had evolved from the politely curious small talk, "Do you have children?" into the more insistent and urgent demand, "*Why* don't you have any children?"

"Because I haven't been able to have kids yet."

Not that it's any of your business, I thought.

"Are you barren?" he asked.

Does anyone use that antiquated word anymore? I wondered. Apparently they did. It conjured up images in my mind of a dry, desolate wasteland.

"I prefer the term *trying to conceive*," I said.

I'd had difficulty in conceiving, but I hadn't seen myself as "barren" or even "infertile."

I took the lollipops anyway.

As I left the bank, I was reminded of the scene in the movie *Raising Arizona* where H. I. and Edwina "Ed" McDunnough are informed that she is infertile: "And the doc went on to explain that this woman, who looked as fertile as the Tennessee Valley, could bear no young. Her insides were a rocky place where my seed could find no purchase."

Throughout the ages, the names for women living with infertility have been unflattering. Some of the oldest human civilizations arose in a region known as the "Cradle of Civilization" or the "Fertile Crescent." These ancient societies worshipped deities that were associated with agriculture, as well as with human fertility, sex, pregnancy, and childbirth. For thousands of years, fertility rites involving animal sacrifices to gods and goddesses were performed in the Fertile Crescent to encourage fertility in both crops and women. At this time, fertility in women and fertility in agriculture were inseparable, which was reflected in the names for childless women that compared them metaphorically to infertile land. The Akkadian word for a celibate nun was "abandoned field" (*naditu*). The Hebrew word for an infertile woman was "desolate" (*galmuda*), which also meant "stony field" in Arabic. In the ancient Greek world, infertility was described as *apharos*, meaning "nonbearing," but also "unplowed, untilled." Latin gave us "sterile" (*sterilitas*), which could refer to the inability of land to produce crops and also to a woman's inability to reproduce. The bleak-sounding "barren" goes back to the Middle Ages and is derived from the Old French *baraigne*, meaning nonbearing, unproductive, and unfruitful. "Barren" originally meant anything that was incapable of producing its own kind, from plants to animals; it later referred to women as well, but not men.

Such uncomplimentary names reflect negative perceptions of infertility, especially in women. As we've seen, wives of the past might be divorced or discarded for not bearing children. A childless woman may be cast out of her family, shunned by society, or even burned at the stake as a witch. History has many unfavorable tropes of unmarried women without children who were ridiculed and mocked in satirical poems, plays, and ballads. She was characterized as a crone, a hag, an old maid, or a spinster, suggesting a tragic older woman left on the shelf. In stark contrast, an unmarried, childless man is a *bachelor*, which has positive connotations of youth and vigor. One of the first recorded usages of the word is in Geoffrey Chaucer's *Canterbury Tales*, in which the twenty-year-old Squire is described as "a lover and lusty bacheler" who spends his time dancing, singing, and chasing women. A bachelor is eligible, but a spinster is not.

Modern society still judges women who, either intentionally or unintentionally, don't have children. They are viewed with pity, shame, and discomfort. This powerful stigma is reflected in the language of infertility, which is shrouded in shame and blame. Women without children are still branded childless, sterile, and barren, words that imply a woman is somehow inadequate, inferior, and a worthless member of society. Her infertility is seen as a sign of personal or moral failing. She is talked about as being physically deficient, defective, and broken. The medical industry doesn't help with this portrayal, favoring cold, clinical terms like infecund, involuntarily childless, and of course, infertile.

I favored the term "trying to conceive" because it sounded proactive and empowering. But, since my surgery, another six months had gone by without success, and while we were definitely still trying to conceive, I was beginning to accept that I was unable to conceive, without some help.

I was infertile.

Troubleshooting

"It's strange that they're called 'fertility clinics' when they're for people with *infertility*," Matt observed.

"I suppose that's because they aim to make infertile people fertile," I said.

Yet again, it was back to the doctor's office for us, but it was finally time to visit a reproductive endocrinologist. I hadn't even heard of reproductive endocrinology until Dr. Schwarz had talked about it with us just six months before. You don't just wake up one morning and decide to go to a fertility clinic. It's a gradual process, taken one step at a time. It had been a long road for us to get to this point, a journey that was hindered by hurdles and delays. There is a kind of stagnation to infertility. Nurses, doctors, and surgeons had told us to "just wait and see." We'd been given lots of advice along the way, both good and bad, and sometimes we'd been cast adrift without any advice at all. This is a common path for many people, who are not referred to a specialist soon enough. When we finally got to this place, we felt beaten down, but we still had a steep hill to climb. I wish I'd known then what I knew now. At first, we didn't even know if we were infertile, and we didn't want to be branded with that label because it felt like giving up. Over time we realized that acknowledging our infertility was actually empowering. It was the beginning of finding a solution. It's like troubleshooting, or problem-solving, to find the root cause of the infertility to then (hopefully) restore fertility.

Having now taken on the label of infertility myself, it was time to revisit what this means according to the medical industry. The technical definition of infertility is the inability to conceive after having frequent and unprotected sex for one year or more. For those over thirty-five, this time frame is reduced to six months. But in reality, it can take a lot longer than six months or even a year to figure out there's something wrong. Infertility is also a lot broader than this simplistic definition, and it can also mean the ability to get pregnant but then suffering miscarriages and stillbirths. As noted previously, there are two types of infertility: primary infertility, when a pregnancy or live birth has never been achieved, and secondary infertility, which is the inability to become pregnant or carry a baby to term after previously giving birth.

There is much debate over whether infertility is a disease or not. It was only a few years ago that the World Health Organization officially defined it as such. It is a disorder of the reproductive system; however, it is not given the recognition it deserves. Infertility is often classified as "unexplained" because there is no known reason for it, and in the absence of physical manifestations, it can be considered a type of hidden disability. It is a serious medical condition, although it is widely discriminated against by society and by the medical and insurance industries, which largely ignore infertility, deeming it something minor or frivolous. Uncharitably, some people consider infertility with underlying conditions to be "real" or "genuine," meanwhile criticizing others who suffer it for simply being "too old" or "waiting too long" to have children. As we know, women are seen as irresponsible for having kids "too early," but also for "leaving it too late." However, infertility is infertility, and no particular type or cause is more or less legitimate or valid. We should encourage a sisterhood of infertility, having empathy and showing support for those who suffer alongside us, because infertility is difficult enough without infighting.

The very first fertility clinic was the Sterility Clinic, founded in 1926 by obstetrician and gynecologist John Rock in Brookline, Massachusetts. (Rock is best known for his role in developing the birth control pill.) Today there are about five hundred fertility clinics and almost two thousand reproductive endocrinologists in the US alone. After careful consideration, we decided to visit a local fertility clinic in Denver, because it was convenient and had a good reputation. From the list of doctors, we chose to see Dr. Wynn, whose online biography described her as "caring and compassionate." We had to wait several months for our appointment—demand is high because many couples and individuals struggle with infertility. An estimated 15 percent of couples will have trouble conceiving. More than one hundred million individuals suffer from infertility worldwide. These figures are on the rise, with some doctors and researchers saying infertility is becoming an epidemic. This is possibly because more people are waiting to have children, while there is also more of a focus on the issue than there has ever been. On the bright side, because of this, there are now more medical advances and treatment options.

We waited nervously in Dr. Wynn's office. Her room was decorated with framed photographs of adorable twins in Anne

Geddes–style poses. Like trophies hanging on the walls, these were the babies born to their patients, the clinic's success stories. The sight was both heartening and a kick to the gut. As I felt tears well up in my eyes, I noticed there were tissue boxes within reach in every room of the clinic. I grabbed a few tissues and stuffed them into my pockets.

"Good morning," trilled Dr. Wynn as she breezed into the office and took her seat. "What are we here for today?"

What do you think we're here for?! I thought.

"Infertility," I replied.

We gave her an overview of our long story. Prior to our appointment, we had also completed an extensive medical history, detailing our family tree of reproductive health, including that of our parents, grandparents, and even our siblings. We were asked embarrassing questions about STDs, sexuality, whether we drink or take drugs, and how many times a week we have unprotected sex. Baby-making is usually such a private matter, but when you're infertile, your personal health, history, and sex life are laid bare. It feels like an invasion of privacy, but it is a necessary one if you seek help.

"We're going to do some day 3 testing," said Dr. Wynn. "We'll check your AMH, FSH, LH, and E2," she said, rattling off a bunch of mostly unfamiliar abbreviations. It's annoying when doctors expect you to understand their lingo without explaining it.

"What happens next?" I asked.

"Call when you start your next period."

I'd just menstruated, so we would have to wait another month before we could move forward. Time is never experienced so intensely as when you're infertile.

"It was nice to meet you both," said Dr. Wynn as she shook our hands and breezed out of the office.

We sat alone in the room again, except for the twin babies on the walls.

"That was it?" asked Matt.

"I guess so," I replied, thinking the doctor was less caring and compassionate and more indifferent.

At the first sign of my next period I called the clinic, and Nurse Kim scheduled me to come in on cycle day 3 to have my blood drawn for a range of fertility tests. Anti-Mullerian levels, or AMH, measure the size of ovarian reserve, or the egg count. Follicle stimulating hormone, or FSH, is produced by the pituitary gland in the brain. As the name suggests, the hormone is responsible for growing the follicles that hold eggs each menstrual cycle and getting one egg ready for ovulation. Luteinizing hormone, or LH, is also produced by the pituitary gland. As stated in chapter 2, its role is to regulate the length of the menstrual cycle and trigger the release of a mature follicle. LH is lower at the beginning of a period and surges right before ovulation. That's why many ovulation tests measure this hormone to help pinpoint when ovulation is approaching. Estradiol, or E2, is a hormone produced by the ovaries and also by the placenta during pregnancy. It plays many roles, including kick-starting the process that leads to ovulation. For women of reproductive age, these hormone levels fluctuate not only day-to-day but also hour-to-hour. The reason these tests are done on day 3 of the menstrual cycle is that this is considered to be the "baseline," when the levels of reproductive hormones are most stable, before they begin to rise.

I was anxious to receive my test results. A few days later I got a phone call from Kim.

"Your levels were all within range," she announced.

I breathed a sigh of relief.

"Although your AMH was what we call 'low normal,'" she added.

A high AMH means a higher number of eggs than is expected for one's age (which is often a sign of PCOS. High levels of AMH can stop an egg from being released even if it's ready.). A low AMH is an indication of a decreased egg reserve, and means that time for conception is running out. Low normal means on the low end of the acceptable range. That my AMH was low normal was to be expected, given that one of my ovaries was much smaller than average.

"What do we do next?" I asked.

"The doctor suggests you try a series of IUIs," replied Kim.

I remembered that Dr. Moore had predicted that we might have to try intrauterine insemination, or IUI. I was excited by the thought of finally getting some professional help.

"Let's do it."

"Great!" she said. "Call when you start your next period."

The Turkey Baster Method

"We're going to use a turkey baster?" Matt joked.

"Not exactly," I replied, rolling my eyes.

The famed "turkey baster method" refers to artificial insemination, or as doctors call it, intracervical insemination (ICI). "Turkey baster" is an allusion to the tool used in cooking, a plastic tube attached to a rubber bulb, that's made to suck up juices from a pan to pour over meat. The technique involves delivering sperm into the reproductive tract, right near the cervical opening, which is the doorway to the uterus. The goal is to improve the chances of fertilization by increasing the number of sperm that reach the fallopian tubes when the woman is most fertile. Insemination is functionally the same thing as sexual intercourse, except instead of using a penis to inseminate, a tool is used. While repurposing a turkey baster is certainly possible, many couples prefer to use one of the commercially available disposable syringes. There are many scenarios in which people try this type of at-home insemination. A "home job" is often preferred by same-sex couples who are ready to start their family, and by people who want to parent without a partner, including single mothers by choice. It's also helpful for those with erectile dysfunction, people with physical disabilities, or those who opt to use donor sperm. This is an attractive option for many people because they can inseminate in the comfort and privacy of their own home.

In contrast to intracervical insemination, which puts sperm near the cervix, intrauterine insemination involves placing sperm directly into the uterus, getting them even closer to the egg to avoid many of the hurdles of their journey. IUI is performed at a clinic by a doctor or nurse, not done in the home. While ICI requires a healthy sperm specimen, IUI can bypass problems with sperm quality, quantity, and movement. This is because the sample undergoes a "sperm wash," in which the healthy, swimming sperm are separated from the rest and a solution containing antibiotics and proteins is added to the ejaculate before it is inseminated. IUI is a great option for those who have a healthy uterus, at least one working ovary, and at least one fallopian tube that is open. Most patients will undergo a hysterosalpingogram (HSG) or saline infusion sonogram (SIS) to ensure that this is the case, but I'd already undergone a dye test as part of my laparoscopy. Some patients choose to have an "unstimulated" or natural cycle of IUI, while others have a "stimulated" cycle, which involves taking fertility drugs such as oral tablets or injectables. I was prescribed a mild fertility drug at the beginning of my period. Ironically, I was placed on Clomid, the same medication Matt had taken to improve his sperm. Women who have irregular or infrequent periods take Clomid for ovulation induction, but it can also be used to stimulate the ovaries to produce multiple egg follicles. With only one normal ovary, I needed all the help I could get.

Timing is crucial when it comes to IUI, to synchronize the insemination with ovulation. To this end, some women take a "trigger shot" of the pregnancy hormone human gonadotrophin (HCG) to stimulate the release of the egg(s). I was monitored closely with transvaginal ultrasounds, in which a probe is placed inside the vagina to measure my follicles as they grew. I also had blood work every few days to check my LH levels so clinic staff could determine the best time for my procedure. But there is no consensus on the optimal timing of IUI. It is an inexact science. They are performed "around" the time the egg is released from the ovary, typically eighteen to thirty-six hours after the LH surge is detected. We were doing a single insemination attempt, whereas some couples undergo double inseminations around the time of ovulation to try to catch that elusive egg. As we know, sperm can survive in the reproductive tract for up to three days, although the egg lasts less than twenty-four hours. Others follow up an IUI with good old-fashioned sexual intercourse. This is crudely called a "sperm chaser," named after the bartending term for a weaker drink taken after a shot of hard liquor.

The day of my IUI, we arrived two hours ahead of the procedure to allow for a sperm sample to be collected and washed in the laboratory to concentrate the sperm and remove the seminal fluid. (Seminal fluid can cause severe cramping in the uterus due to the effects of prostaglandin, a hormone-like substance in sperm to which some people are sensitive. We might remember that prostaglandins also cause menstrual cramps.) In the exam room, we were dismayed to discover that our sperm count was slightly lower than normal.

"But it only takes one sperm!" enthused Nurse Kim, who was performing the insemination.

Her positive attitude allayed our fears.

I had to have a full bladder before the procedure, to facilitate the insertion of the catheter. As I lay on an examination table with my legs up in the stirrups and a speculum in my vagina, she guided a catheter through my cervical opening and into my uterus. It felt similar to having a Pap smear and was a little uncomfortable, but this was still nowhere near as invasive as IVF.

"Ready?" she asked.

I took a deep breath.

"Yes."

Matt held my hand and looked into my eyes as the sperm sample was injected into me. This wasn't the most sexy or romantic attempt at making a baby, but it was significantly increasing our chances of pregnancy.

"All done!" said Kim.

"That's it?" I asked.

"Yes," she replied. "But I want you to stay lying down for fifteen minutes."

Contrary to the common misconception, there's no need to remain prone after intercourse or IUI to keep the sperm inside the body (the cervix doesn't remain open), but studies show that lying flat for ten to twenty minutes after IUI increases the likelihood of pregnancy compared with moving around afterward. After this time, I could also empty my bursting bladder, although some swear that holding on for up to an hour improves their chances.

"You may experience some bleeding and cramping afterward, but that's normal," warned Kim. "Good luck, and I'll see you in two weeks for your pregnancy test!"

That was easy, I thought.

Now came the hard part.

Waiting.

But after all of the urban legends and folk medicine I'd tried, I was excited to be trying some science.

Something in the Water

When infertility was no longer considered a punishment for sin, a curse, or an evil spell cast by a witch, it became recognized as a physical condition, and one that was possibly reversible. But in the past, medical science wasn't always very scientific. Early Greek physicians experimented with various surgical interventions, inflating the uterus or dilating it with hollow lead probes to remove any "blockages," but often causing infertility in the process. To cure a "wandering womb," honey, perfumed oils, and other sweet substances were applied to the vagina to lure the uterus back into place. The Greek physician Aretaeus of Cappadocia wrote, "The womb delights in fragrant smells and advances towards them; but it has an aversion to fetid smells, and flees from them." Similarly, to drive the womb away from the upper parts of the body, foul-smelling substances were introduced to the nostrils, including cow dung and "oisype," soiled wool from a goat's anus.

Vaginal suppositories were a popular treatment for infertility. A Babylonian cure says, "To make a not bearing-child woman pregnant you flay an edible mouse, open it up and fill it with myrrh. You dry it in the shade, crush it, grind it up and mix it with fat. You place it in her vagina and she will become pregnant." As we've seen, "kitchen physic" for barrenness was popular in almanacs and domestic remedy books. One medical recipe from the fifteenth century advises soaking a pad in a solution made of oil and the powdered right testicle of a weasel and placing it in the vagina as a pessary. Sympathetic magic was still popular, and animal testicles and penises were used widely in fertility treatments. Another home remedy says an infertile woman should "drink several compounds of boiled pine twigs and white wine, and of celery, cumin seed and frankincense, accompanied by eating boiled puppy and octopus, and bathing twice a day." These animals were chosen for their fertile reputation; puppies are born in litters, while an octopus can have over fifty thousand babies at one time.

In the Middle Ages, bleeding and leeches were cure-alls that were also used to treat infertility. As we've seen, if an infertile woman was "corpulent," she was told to purge or sweat out her excess weight with hot sand or steam baths. "Taking the waters" at fertility towns—that is, bathing in or sometimes even drinking their spa waters—was also believed to benefit fertility. There are many tales of its apparent success. Queen Mary II visited the hot springs of Bath and became pregnant ten months later. King Charles I's consort Henrietta Maria was wooed by the hot springs in Welling-borough, and she fell pregnant soon afterward. It's said she kept a medicine chest by her bed that was full of fertility waters collected from around the UK, and she went on to have nine children. The baths also developed a reputation for sexual scandal. The 1658 poem "Upon a Lady that went to Tunbridge Wells" tells the story of a woman who was cured of her sterility at the bath, not by the waters, but by the intervention of "a lusty cock of the game." But the waters didn't seem to help everyone. Henrietta's daughter-in-law, Catherine of Braganza, tried the waters at Tunbridge Wells, but she produced no heirs, having suffered three miscarriages, although her husband Charles II fathered at least twelve illegitimate children. To this day, people visit fertility towns to take the waters in the hopes of getting pregnant. During the filming of the movie *Australia*, Nicole Kidman became pregnant unexpectedly at the age of forty-one after swimming in the waterfalls in the outback town of Kunnunurra, Western Australia. A total of seven babies were conceived during the filming of the movie, which the film crew attributed to the "fertility waters."

Some enterprising individuals invented gadgets and contraptions to aid in conception. Scotsman James Graham was an eighteenth-century pioneer in sex therapy. A self-styled doctor, he was best known for his "Celestial Bed," designed for couples struggling with infertility. The bed was reserved for those willing and able to afford the fee of fifty pounds per night (which in modern US dollars amounts to over $5,000.) The bed was "powered" by magnets, and "Dr." Graham advertised that anyone who rented the bed was guaranteed "immediate conception." The magical bed was twelve feet long by nine wide and could be tilted for use at various angles. The mattress was stuffed with oat straw mingled with lavender flowers and covered with silk damask. The air was perfumed with roses and "oriental spices." As lovers lay in bed, they listened to the soft orchestral music playing in the distance and could stare up into a large mirror suspended above them on the ceiling. The words "Be fruitful. Multiply, and replenish the Earth" were inscribed on the headboard.

Other devices were popular for curing infertility, such as those used for vaginal fumigation. An ancient Egyptian recipe says, "You should fumigate her with spelt in her vagina until it ceases, to allow for her husband's seed to be received." Fumigation involved using an apparatus that introduced herb-infused steam or smoke into the woman's vagina. This technique was later advocated by Hippocrates and remained in vogue for centuries. According to *The Trotula*, infertility was caused by an imbalance of the humors. Once the temperature of a woman's womb was established, it was recommended that her vagina be fumigated with herbs of the opposite temperature. If she was too hot, she should use "marsh mallows, violets, and roses in water," while if she was too cold, she should try "clove, spikenard, and nutmeg." In modern times, vaginal fumigation has made a comeback. Actress and influencer Gwyneth Paltrow has promoted a contraption called the "V Steam." As she put it: "You sit on what is essentially a mini-throne, and a combination of infrared and mugwort steam cleanses your uterus." Paltrow advocates the practice for vaginal hygiene, while the company claims that it works for infertility too, although medical professionals don't recommend it.

There were few medical options for infertility until the late twentieth century and the advent of what are called assisted reproductive technologies (ART). These include IUI and IVF. Today, IUI is the first-line fertility treatment, because it's not as expensive or invasive as IVF. Artificial insemination has a long history. We might remember Henry "the Impotent," the fifteenth-century king of Castile, and the rumors that his daughter Juana was the product of his wife's infidelity. Unofficial history claims that the princess was actually conceived via artificial insemination. We might also remember that in the late 1700s, Italian priest Lazzaro Spallanzani successfully inseminated fish, frogs, and dogs. The first successful artificial insemination of a woman was recorded just one decade later, when Scottish surgeon John Hunter helped a linen draper's wife to get pregnant with her husband's sperm. The couple was having difficulties because he suffered from severe hypospadias (just like King Henry II of France and his "malformed penis"). To perform the insemination, semen that escaped during sex was collected into a warmed syringe and injected into the woman's vagina, which resulted in pregnancy and a live birth. Hundreds of years later, IUI is a very popular procedure used by many worldwide.

Today's methods for treating infertility are more scientific than the science of the past, but that isn't to say that success is guaranteed.

Don't Count Your Chickens Before They Hatch

It was two weeks post-IUI, the timeframe known as the agonizing "two-week wait," and I was sitting in the clinic waiting for my pregnancy test. There was no sign of my period yet, so I was cautiously optimistic. With great willpower I had avoided the allure of the "pee on a stick" (or "POAS") pregnancy tests and had waited patiently for the definitive blood test. As mentioned before, HCG is a hormone produced in the body during pregnancy. The quantitative HCG test measures the specific level of this hormone in the blood. A positive test means pregnancy, while the number indicates how far along a woman is in her pregnancy. At this point, I would be around two weeks pregnant. I kept a stoic face while the nurse punctured my arms repeatedly in her search for a vein. Afterward, I was told I'd be contacted with the test results that afternoon. I left the office with neon orange-colored bandages wrapped around both arms. As I exited the building, I heard a loud chirping sound above in an aspen tree. I looked up and spotted a mother bird in a nest feeding her baby chicks. I took this as a positive sign.

Birds have a more interesting reproductive system than we might think. Male birds have two testes, while females have two ovaries. Both sexes have one on the right and one on the left. However, most female birds have only one working ovary. The evolutionary loss of one functional ovary was a weight-saving change that may have proved beneficial to flying birds. Some birds have interesting sex lives too. After a rooster inseminates a hen, her eggs can be fertilized for up to four weeks. This is because the sperm remains viable for this time, stored in "sperm nests" in the hen's oviduct. On the other hand, many chickens don't have sex lives at all. Most hens raised in commercial farms are virgins, and they don't need roosters in order to lay eggs. (In a process known as parthenogenesis, a form of procreation among ants, bees, and some birds, an egg can develop into an embryo without being fertilized by sperm, resulting in a "virgin birth.") The only thing hens need in order to stimulate egg-laying is light. Hens are programmed to lay eggs in the spring and summer, which they judge by the amount of daylight.

Commercial farmers exploit this tendency by simulating summer days in their chicken coops all year round. Chickens are egg-laying machines. A hen hits puberty just months after hatching out of an egg herself. It only takes a day for her to make an egg, and then she can start to produce another just one hour later. Impressively, hens lay up to three hundred eggs every year.

If a bird can have babies with only one ovary, then so can I, I thought.

I sat at home waiting for the phone call. As I did, I googled success rates for artificial insemination. The pregnancy statistics for ICI are slightly lower than for IUI, with home insemination resulting in 9 percent success per cycle, while insemination performed at a clinic results in 15 percent per cycle. These rates were low, but better than my chances without help. And the statistics increase with multiple attempts. The cumulative pregnancy rate for ICI is 37.9 percent after six treatment cycles, while there is a 40.5 percent success rate for IUI after six treatments. Of course, these success rates are affected by many different factors, such as the cause of infertility, the age of the patients, and whether donor sperm is used or not.

When my phone finally rang, I nearly jumped out of my skin. It was Kim.

My heart sank when I could tell by the tone of her voice that the news was not good.

"Your HCG levels were less than 5," she said. "I'm sorry."

An HCG level of less than 5 mIU/ml (milli-international units per milliliter) is considered negative for pregnancy, while anything above 25 mIU/ml is considered positive for pregnancy. I was part of the 85 percent of people who do not get pregnant on the first IUI attempt.

"But there's always the next cycle!" said Kim, trying to remain positive. "Call when you get your next period."

This seemed to be the mantra of the fertility clinic.

I hung up the phone, feeling like a bucket of ice water had been thrown over me.

For Sale: Baby Shoes, Never Worn

My period started the next day.

I took a mental health day away from work and curled up in front of the TV with a hot water bottle and a cup of tea, but this probably wasn't the best time to watch the movie *Up*. The opening montage begins with childhood sweethearts Carl and Ellie Fredricksen, who vow to embark on adventures together one day. They marry, and dream of their future together, their music-scored dreams including visions of babies. They are shown decorating a nursery and preparing for a baby, but then we see them in a doctor's office. Ellie cries into her hands and her husband consoles her while they face the doctor. Clearly, she suffers infertility or she had had a pregnancy loss. Afterward, we see Ellie sitting alone outside, her eyes closed, as she projects a deep pain and sadness. Years later she passes away, never having had any children.

I sobbed throughout the movie.

Reproductive challenges are among the most trying human conditions. Infertility causes intense sadness and desperation, powerlessness and despair. Every period is a painful reminder month after month that, once again, you're not pregnant. Infertility creates an irreparable sense of loss, as though someone is missing. Former US President George W. Bush and Laura Bush tried to conceive for years, but pregnancy didn't come easy for them. After five years of marriage, the couple had started the adoption process when they discovered they were expecting twins. Laura had grown up as an only child in a family that lost three babies to miscarriage or infant death. In her memoir, she writes eloquently about the grief of infertility:

> The English language lacks the words to mourn an absence. For the loss of a parent, grandparent, spouse, child, or friend, we have all manner of words and phrases, some helpful, some not. Still, we are conditioned to say something, even if it is only "I'm sorry for your loss." But for an absence, for someone who was never there at all, we are wordless to capture that particular emptiness. For those who deeply want children and are denied them, those missing babies hover like silent, ephemeral shadows over their lives. Who can describe the feel of a tiny hand that is never held?

The sense of sadness and loss caused by infertility is a common theme in popular culture, literature, and folklore. There is an apocryphal story about Ernest Hemingway, that during lunch with fellow writers one day, he made a ten-dollar bet with them that he could write a six-word short story. He won the wager when he penned the gut-wrenching words, "For sale: baby shoes, never worn." These six simple words resonate with the heartbreak of infertility and pregnancy loss. However, the attribution is false; the story first emerged many years before Hemingway even began writing, although, sadly, the tale may have been inspired by a true story. In a 1910 edition of *The Spokane Press*, there was an article titled "Tragedy of Baby's Death Is Revealed in Sale of Clothing." The piece recounts an advertisement that struck the author as poignant. The ad read: "Baby's hand made trousseau and baby's bed for sale. Never been used." The writer remarked, "This perhaps meant little to the casual reader, yet to the mother who had spent hours and days planning the beautiful things for her tiny baby, it meant a keen sorrow and disappointment."

Infertility is unfair. Going through the process of accepting the diagnosis drags you through a turbulent cavalcade of emotions: shock, disappointment, self-blame, denial, anger. You inevitably ask yourself painful questions: Why is this happening to me? What did I do to deserve this? Why is my body failing me? Am I not meant to be a mother? But there are no answers to these questions. Injustices seem to play out all around us in news stories of horrific child abuse and neglect. It seems as though so many people have *unwanted* children without any difficulty, while others desperately *want* to have children, but can't. In *Up*, infertility rears its head again later in the movie when Carl encounters Russell, an eight-year-old boy whose father has abandoned him. Carl eventually takes on the role of surrogate grandfather, going with him on the kinds of adventures he'd hoped to have with his wife and child. It's hard to not feel bitterness when some parents don't appreciate their children, while other people are unable to build a family.

In the TV series *Ally McBeal*, the main character, Ally, is haunted by recurring hallucinations of a "dancing baby," a metaphor for the ticking of her biological clock. Once you hear that biological clock ticking, the matter of fertility becomes inescapable. Reproduction is a fact of life, and it is everywhere. It's impossible to scroll through social media without seeing a baby announcement or a sonogram image. We're surrounded by friends, family, colleagues, and even strangers who are pregnant, seemingly without effort, or those who already have babies or children. It's difficult to not feel the sting of jealousy when attending baby showers, visiting friends who've just given birth, or attending children's birthday parties and other social situations involving pregnant women, mothers, and kids—and it's okay to feel envy; it's a normal human emotion.

Some friends may feel guilt at their own fertility and, in their discomfort, may actively exclude infertile friends from social events. It's an unfortunate reality that not all friendships will survive intact. Some may become casualties of infertility. Mother's Day, Father's Day, and other family holidays are times of sadness and emptiness. Everything seems to be a reminder of infertility, from diaper commercials to "Baby on Board" bumper stickers. But while pregnancy and motherhood are visible and celebrated, infertility is often invisible and silent. With some 15 percent of people living with infertility, we're not alone. But while there is a certain camaraderie to infertility, it also brings a deep sense of loneliness. An infertile woman feels like the odd one out. She is separated from pregnant women and mothers, and isolated from society in general, feeling like she doesn't fit in or belong anywhere.

Infertility negatively affects quality of life and health, especially mental health. Depression and anxiety are common among people living with infertility, leading them to feel out of control, helpless, sad, fearful, frustrated, and worried all the time. This trauma can occasionally lead to extreme behavior. Phantom pregnancy, or pseudocyesis, is a phenomenon in which a hopeful mom-to-be believes she's pregnant and may even have the physical symptoms to back it up, but she's not actually expecting a baby. In these cases, when there's a desperate yearning for pregnancy, the mind has a surprisingly powerful influence on the body, generating pregnancy symptoms when there's no actual baby growing. A famous example is that of Mary Tudor, daughter of Henry VIII and Katherine of Aragon. Aged thirty-seven and unmarried when she became queen, Mary was anxious to secure her throne with an heir, just like her father had been all those years before. She married quickly and soon showed signs of pregnancy; her periods stopped, she suffered morning sickness, she gained weight, and she even felt the "quickening," the baby's movements in the womb. But after almost a year of symptoms, the child failed to materialize, and it became clear that Mary was not pregnant. A few years later it happened again, but this time whatever illness plagued her proved to be fatal. Modern historians speculate that these were false pregnancies, or that she suffered from ovarian, uterine, or stomach cancer. Mary's prayer book has survived, which still shows evidence of tear stains on the page containing the "Prayer for Expectant Mothers."

In rare cases, women go to extreme lengths to get a baby. Some have been driven to steal a newborn baby from a hospital or from a new mother. There have been hundreds of child abductions in the United States over the past few decades, as well as recorded cases from many countries across Europe, Asia, South America, and Australia. A gruesome example is fetal abduction by maternal evisceration, which happens when a woman desires a baby so badly that she attacks a mother-to-be and cuts the baby from the womb, then passes it off as her own. The perpetrators, sometimes derisively dubbed "womb raiders," usually feign a pregnancy, stealing another woman's sonograms and even setting up a registry for friends to buy them baby gifts. They target a friend, acquaintance, or stranger and make plans to steal a full-term fetus, often luring the victim with the promise of baby clothes. In one case, a woman taught herself how to conduct a caesarean section by watching a TV show on the Discovery Channel. The mothers-to-be and babies rarely survive the ordeal. It must be strongly stated that this behavior is not a normal response to fertility problems. These offenders have serious psychological issues, and their actions are therefore *not* motivated by infertility.

Such sad stories reminded me again of the movie *Raising Arizona*, in which H. I. and Ed are desperate to have a child, but she is infertile. They discover that local furniture magnate Nathan Arizona's wife, Florence, has just birthed quintuplet sons (implying that the infants were a result of assisted reproductive technologies). In a reckless move, the couple kidnaps one of the babies, Nathan Jr. At the movie's end, they finally return the baby to his relieved father, Nathan Sr. In her defense, Ed says, "We didn't want to hurt him any. I just wanted to be a mama." Nathan Sr. asks them, "Just tell me why you did it." H. I. admits, "We can't have one of our own." The man replies, "If you can't have kids, you just gotta keep trying and hope medical science catches up with you, like Florence and me. It caught up with a vengeance." That night, H.I. dreams of "an old couple being visited by their children and all their grandchildren too"—the implication being the happy ending that these were *their* children and grandchildren.

These stories of child kidnappings, whether fictional or true-life, ultimately do a disservice to people with infertility. Some women report their friends remarking, "I'd better hide my children from you!" with these stories in mind. Such attitudes are hurtful and ignorant. Those with infertility do not want to be compared or connected to these horrific cases, even in a tangential way. It's the kind of thing that has stigmatized infertility.

Labels like "barren" have also tarnished infertility. Today there is a movement to reclaim the once-dreaded word. Instead of passively accepting "barren" and its negative connotations, some women have reappropriated it as an empowering identity label. But for others the label is factually incorrect. "Barren" implies that a woman can *never* have children, but maybe the truth is that she is only yet to have children. Perhaps barrenness is just a perspective. In the Bible, Sarah, Rebekah, and Rachel were described as "barren," but only because they hadn't had children at that point. They were still trying to conceive, and they eventually did so. Maybe someone who is deemed "infertile" is not permanently so. For this reason, "subfertility," the term used by Dr. Schwarz, is better, because it implies only reduced fertility, not barrenness. It means that trying to conceive is taking longer than expected or hoped for, but that it's not impossible. Perhaps infertility is only a point in the journey, not the journey's end.

From the challenges of infertility, strength emerges. Infertility teaches us to become resilient, persistent, and tough.

I finally understood that while another period was a failure, it was also another chance at success. We were ready to try again.

I called the clinic.

The Last Resort

The next six months were a roller coaster ride. We had ups and downs, feeling hopeful and optimistic one day, then pessimistic the next.

We were excited to try another IUI.

"If at first you don't succeed, try, try again!" said Kim, cheering us on.

We underwent the second round of IUI with a positive attitude, but we were devastated when that failed too, although we weren't going to give up yet.

"Third time's the charm!" Kim enthused.

So we attempted a third round of IUI.

This was around the time that, in my anxiety, I caved in and began using home pregnancy tests. "Using" makes it sound like an addiction, which it can quickly become. When you're trying to get pregnant, every test can feel like a do-or-die situation. A recent study shows that "pee on a stick" addiction is real. More than $200 million is spent on pregnancy tests every year. Self-described "POAS addicts" test compulsively, spending hundreds of dollars to test for pregnancy month after month, and even continuing to test obsessively *after* doctors have confirmed a pregnancy.

The ritual of testing only added to the stress for me, because our third round was also unsuccessful. Then our fourth, fifth, *and sixth* attempts failed too. The cumulative effects of multiple IUI cycles didn't work for us. By this time, we were mentally and emotionally exhausted. Over the years, infertility had hijacked our lives. Through timed intercourse and now IUIs, we had been living at the mercy of my menstrual cycle. Our pursuit of pregnancy had become all-consuming. We were going around in circles and didn't know what to do next. We weren't sure if we should attempt a seventh IUI or just go back to trying to conceive naturally. Completely demoralized, we were summoned back to the clinic to see Dr. Wynn. Walking through the waiting room, we passed by a couple sitting on a couch, their eyes red and swollen from crying. It was like we were staring into a mirror.

In Dr. Wynn's office it seemed as though the portraits of twins on the walls had multiplied since our last visit.

"It's nice to see you again," she said, motioning for us to sit down.

To be honest, we'd felt abandoned by Dr. Wynn during our IUI cycles. It seemed as though Nurse Kim had done all of the hard work.

"We're here today to discuss your failed IUI cycles," she said.

The word "failed" stung, although it was true.

"Should we try another IUI?" I asked.

"You've already had *six* cycles of IUIs," she replied curtly. "That's the recommended amount for your age."

If no pregnancy occurs after six rounds of IUI, most people call it quits and move on to something else. When it comes to fertility treatments, you always need to have the next strategy lined up. When something doesn't work, you need to have a Plan B.

"Should we go back to trying again naturally?" asked Matt.

"Your chances of conceiving naturally are a mere 1 percent," she said, again curtly. "At this point, your *only* chance at success is to try IVF."

I felt a ripple of fear run through my body. In vitro fertilization had always seemed like the last resort, but here we were.

"How much will that cost?" I asked.

Infertility is not only a psychological and social burden, but also a financial one. Cost is an important consideration for most people. We'd already spent thousands of dollars on IUIs, paid out-of-pocket without any support from our insurance company, not to mention the expense of all the previous diagnostic work and surgeries.

"I recommend you have IVF with ICSI and PGS," she said, again expecting us to magically understand specialized medical terminology. "That's going to cost about this much." She scribbled a figure on a notepad and tore off the page. With a strange smile on her face, she thrust the paper across the table. The quote was for a very high five-figure sum.

"Not including medications," she added. "And of course, there are still no guarantees that it will work."

We felt helpless and hopeless.

Seeing tears well up in my eyes, Dr. Wynn slid the ubiquitous box of tissues toward me.

"I'll let you think about it," she said, before breezing out of her office.

Left alone in the silent room, we suddenly became aware of the ticking sound coming from the clock on the wall.

7

TEST-TUBE BABIES

In Vitro Fertilization

"I want to try IVF," I said.

I had reached the point where I not only wanted to try IVF, but was also resigned to the fact that we needed to do so. I was disappointed, nervous, and excited, all at once.

"Let's try it," agreed Matt. "But not with them."

Our first experience with a fertility clinic had not been ideal. Our reproductive endocrinologist had a bad bedside manner—that is, on those few occasions we actually saw her. The clinic had good success rates, but we soon learned that a doctor shouldn't be chosen based on percentages alone. (Many clinics purport to have "one of the highest success rates in the nation!") So we searched around the city, state, and country, doing our research and reading reviews. We visited another clinic, then another, and yet another.

The doctors we encountered in our search were at times arrogant, condescending, or unsympathetic, and made us wait a long time to be seen, only to spend little time with us. IVF is an intimate experience, and we wanted to find a trustworthy clinic with which we felt comfortable. It was important for us to find a doctor who not only gave us confidence in them, but who also showed they had confidence in us. So-called "doctor shopping" is usually frowned upon by doctors and insurance companies, but it is part of the process of choosing a fertility clinic, to find one that is a good fit. Clinics should support not only the clinical but also the emotional needs of their patients. And even when you find that clinic that's a good fit, still be prepared for a bumpy ride. When you're dealing with a medical team also assigned to many other patients, there will likely be miscommunication, mistakes, and bad experiences along the way. As fertility patients, we need to advocate for ourselves because no one else will. But we're not just patients; we're also consumers, who have rights to explore our options and make active and informed decisions about our health care.

We did some more searching and finally found another clinic in Denver that sounded promising. It was part of a teaching hospital, which are known for using state-of-the-art treatments and technologies. I called them to schedule an appointment, but we were soon to find out that no experience with any fertility clinic is ever ideal.

"Which doctor would you like to schedule an appointment with?" asked the receptionist.

"Dr. Jones, please," I replied.

"I'm sorry," she said. "Dr. Jones will be going on maternity leave soon."

"That's nice," I heard myself say.

How ironic, I thought. Infertility was inescapable, right down to the reproductive endocrinologist who couldn't be our doctor because *she* was pregnant. I'd discovered, too, that some fertility doctors aren't sympathetic because they haven't suffered infertility themselves and can't relate to it.

"I can recommend Dr. Ross instead," suggested the receptionist. "She's new to our clinic, and she has an opening in two weeks."

"We'll take it," I said.

A few weeks later we arrived for our initial consultation with Dr. Ross. Being part of a hospital, the clinic was comparatively understated, without any framed baby photos on the walls to add to the pressure. It was so discreet it might just as well have been a doctor's office to have an annual physical exam or to get a mole checked.

Dr. Ross ushered us into her office.

"Nice to meet you," she said, shaking our hands warmly.

She had a friendly smile, and we immediately felt at ease with her. "Tell me your story."

We told Dr. Ross about our long journey, all the way up to our experiences at the previous clinics. She listened carefully and nodded in understanding.

"IVF will definitely give you the best chance at pregnancy," she concluded. "You have a 65 percent chance of getting pregnant using IVF, which increases to 75 percent with preimplantation genetic screening. This testing checks your embryos for any chromosomal abnormalities before they are transferred into your uterus."

This was the mysterious "PGS" that our previous doctor had glossed over in her spiel. Some fertility doctors don't entrust patients with knowledge about their health and options, so they are not empowered in any way, just told what to do.

"I must tell you that IVF poses a higher risk of multiples," warned Dr. Ross. "There's a greater likelihood that you might have twins as a result of this treatment."

It seemed incongruous to go from a discussion about not being able to have children *at all* to suddenly talking about the possibility of having "too many." This is because multiple pregnancies are common in IVF treatment. When they discovered we would be trying IVF, our friends joked that we'd have twins. Although it is a myth that IVF *always* results in twins. The odds of having a multiple-gestation pregnancy through IVF are roughly 30 percent. The associated risks are that twins and triplets are usually born preterm, with lower birth weights and a greater chance of congenital disorders, while the odds of life-threatening maternal complications are higher with multiples as well. The end goal of infertility treatment is to give birth to one healthy baby, a singleton as they call this in the industry.

We liked Dr. Ross. She was caring and sincere. We listened to that little voice in the back of our heads that told us she was the right doctor for us.

"We'd like to try IVF with you," I said.

"As soon as possible," added Matt. "We don't have time to lose."

"I understand," said Dr. Ross. "We'll put you on the list for our next available cycle."

"When will that be?" I asked.

"Three months from now," she replied.

More waiting, I sighed.

"We'll need to perform infectious disease screening in the meantime," she said. This involves testing for contagious diseases, such as HIV, hepatitis B and C, syphilis, rubella (German measles), and varicella (chicken pox), to prevent their transmission to parents and newborns. Clinics also test for blood type, and may screen for genetic disorders such as cystic fibrosis and Fragile X syndrome.

"Are you taking a prenatal vitamin?" she asked.

"I am." I'd been taking one for years.

"Good," she said. "Call when you start your next period."

Soon thereafter we had to visit the office again to complete the clinic's consent forms. These were a stack of documents that had to be signed and initialed; it was like signing paperwork on closing day to buy a house. The forms were not only to consent to medical treatment, but also to make legal decisions pertaining to IVF and the "disposition" of genetic material under a variety of circumstances. What happens to any frozen eggs, sperm, or embryos in the event of divorce or death? What happens to any leftover embryos when your family is completed? These are important considerations that have been the subject of numerous legal battles over the decades. Even with a watertight contract in place, assisted reproductive technology laws are complicated and new, with many situations entering uncharted waters. In 2013, actress Sophie Vergara and her then fiancé Nick Loeb conceived two embryos via IVF at a California clinic, which were disused when the couple called off their engagement. A contract signed at the time stipulated that neither partner could do anything with the embryos without the other's consent. Years later, Loeb sued Vergara for custody of the two frozen embryos, which were listed as the plaintiffs, named "Emma and Isabella" in court documents. The lawsuit argued that the embryos were being deprived of their inheritance from a trust by not being born, and asked to "give them the right to live." Loeb planned to have the embryos transferred to a surrogate, but the case was ultimately dismissed.

A Boon for the Barren Woman

Many people think that the "birth" of infertility and its treatment occurred with the emergence of IVF, but as we've seen, that is not the case. Infertility is not a distinctly modern experience; it has been around as long as humans have. Similarly, the beginning of IVF was not in 1978 with the birth of the first "test-tube baby," but began with the trailblazers in reproductive science over the centuries. Before they were called test-tube babies, they were "bottle babies." In the 1930s, American biologist Gregory Pincus conducted research on parthenogenesis (the process that allows birds to have "virgin births") and on in vitro fertilization in rabbits. (*In vitro* comes from the Latin term "in glass.") A journalist soon announced the successful birth of a rabbit after Pincus had fertilized eggs from one female rabbit "in a watch glass" and then implanted the resultant embryo into another rabbit. The story invoked the imagery of Aldous Huxley's *Brave New World*, which had just been published in 1932, in which the author imagined a dystopian future where nearly all humans were incubated in specially designed bottles and grown in endless rows of artificial wombs. The novel was probably inspired by Huxley's friend, geneticist J. B. S. Haldane, who in 1924 described a process called "ectogenesis," in which individuals were created outside of the human body. With all of this scaremongering, Pincus received negative publicity for his controversial research and was fired from his position at the Harvard Biological Institute.

IVF pioneer John Rock, whom we might remember as the founder of the first fertility clinic, then hired Pincus's top researcher, Miriam Menkin. If conception in a watch glass could be made to work in humans as well, Rock exclaimed, "What a boon for the barren woman with closed tubes!" Inspired by these "fatherless rabbits," the team applied the findings to human conception, and in 1944 they fertilized the first human egg in a test tube. Without protocols in place to preserve the embryo, it disappeared, but they managed to replicate the results. The pair published their findings in *Science*, but there were still many skeptics at the time. Decades later, English doctors Robert Edwards and Patrick Steptoe, and nurse Jean Purdy, used laparoscopic surgery to retrieve eggs from women and fertilize them in vitro. Over the years they performed hundreds of embryo transfers that failed. In 1975, they announced the first successful pregnancy from IVF; however, it ended in an ectopic pregnancy. But on July 25, 1978, the team captured the world's attention when they revealed the first successful live birth of an IVF baby, Louise Joy Brown. Her parents, Lesley and John Brown, had been trying to conceive naturally for nine years, but Lesley had blocked fallopian tubes. Louise's birth was hailed as a "miracle" by the world's media, and IVF was celebrated as one of the biggest medical breakthroughs of the century. In 2010, Edwards, as the only surviving research partner, was awarded the Nobel Prize for Medicine for his groundbreaking work.

Since the birth of Louise Brown, an estimated ten million babies have been born as a result of assisted reproductive technologies. IVF is a treatment that enables couples with a range of fertility problems to conceive a child, and also allows single mothers by choice and same-sex couples to have children. It's an obvious fact, but worth emphasizing, that these are babies who would otherwise *not* have been born. Now is the best time to be infertile, if one must be infertile, and IVF has given optimism to countless hopeful parents. IVF is the gold standard of fertility treatment options and the most successful currently available. However, as Dr. Wynn had warned us, there are no guarantees that it will work. Despite the optimistic percentages given to us by Dr. Ross, the national success rates are somewhat lower (although much better than they were in the early days of IVF). Depending on who you talk to, the US average is only 37.8 percent live births per embryo transfer. These rates decline steadily with age. In addition, IVF success rates vary according to the cause of infertility, the number of embryos transferred, whether those embryos were fresh or frozen, the use of supplementary techniques, and the patient's history of previous births and miscarriages. I felt demoralized by these low statistics, although Matt reminded me that these rates are only a gauge.

"Their infertility is not your infertility," he said.

Just Do IVF

"You can always just do IVF," was another "simple" solution offered by people when they learned we were having problems trying to conceive.

But not everyone can.

Over the past few decades there has been a drastic increase in the usage of IVF. However, there are barriers to accessing treatment for many who need it. Racial, ethnic, sexual orientation, geographical, and economic disparities affect access to fertility treatments, especially IVF. Far from being an altruistic field of medicine in which doctors want to help people make babies out of the kindness of their hearts, some look at infertility patients with dollar signs in their eyes. IVF is a global, large-scale commercial business and a lucrative mega-million-dollar industry. The treatment is cost-prohibitive for many people because it is usually very expensive. In some countries, IVF is low-cost, government-funded, or subsidized, like it is under Australia's universal health insurance program called Medicare, and the National Health Service in Great Britain. In comparison, in the United States, the cost of just one cycle of IVF can be anywhere in the range of $10,000 to $60,000 or even more. Unlike other areas of health care, many fertility clinics offer financing, so couples and individuals take out exorbitant loans, or even remortgage their homes, for just a shot at success. Without guarantees, IVF is an expensive gamble. At the time of this writing, very few states require insurance plans to cover infertility. Reproductive endocrinology is the "Wild West" of health care, a field of medicine with little oversight and protection from exploitation, with unbridled profit margins. This situation needs to change. Building a family is a basic human right, and while infertility has finally been recognized as a disease, it is not yet treated as such when it comes to health care, because the treatment is often considered a luxury. As part of a teaching hospital, our clinic was reasonably priced (this being a relative term when talking about IVF), but we still had to exhaust our hard-earned savings to pay for a single cycle.

Another potential obstacle to accessing IVF is age. The very first in vitro human embryo, obtained in 1944 by doctors Rock and Menkin, was created with an egg collected from Mrs. D. D., a thirty-eight-year-old woman. Today, nearly 60 percent of IVF procedures in the US are performed on women who are thirty-five or over. Technically, a woman can get pregnant and bear children up until she enters menopause, even during perimenopause (the transition years before the final menstrual period). However, many fertility clinics discriminate against women based on their age. It's true that the ovaries' ability to create viable eggs declines after the mid-thirties, so the chances of achieving pregnancy via IVF are reduced. In the US, IVF success rates plummet for the forty- to forty-two category, while statistics often don't exist for women older than forty-three. In part, this is because many clinics *refuse* to treat women over the age of forty, if they want to use their own eggs. Donor eggs drastically improve chances of pregnancy, but also drastically increase costs. "Donor" is somewhat of a misnomer. The term implies free, a charitable and altruistic donation, but donor eggs are not given free of charge. They can cost tens of thousands of dollars, including compensation for the donor, a cut for the clinic, and often legal fees and other charges. (Donor sperm also costs money, but at a fraction of the cost of donor eggs, because the latter are harder to source. Sperm donors aren't true donors either; they are also paid for their services.) If using donor eggs, many clinics will continue to see patients up to the age of fifty, although different countries have different laws. Erramatti Mangamma, a woman from India, currently holds the record for being the oldest living mother at the age of seventy-four after conceiving healthy twin girls through IVF, using donor eggs fertilized with her eighty-year-old husband's sperm, following fifty-four years of marriage.

A clinic's refusal to provide treatment on the basis of age puts patients in a double bind when IVF is the *only* treatment that might help them. In the US there isn't an official maximum age for conventional IVF, although most clinics impose restrictions on women between their early and mid-forties. This is ostensibly to safeguard the health of patients, who are at an increased risk of miscarriage and medical complications, but it occasionally smacks of clinics trying to preserve their statistics. A woman doesn't turn into a pumpkin when she hits a certain age, so it's unfair to treat her as an age group rather than an individual; the biological clock can vary greatly from woman to woman. Some countries have more flexible upper age limits for undergoing conventional IVF. In the Czech Republic, the legal limit for women to access treatment is forty-nine. In Greece, Spain, and Estonia the age limit is fifty. In Slovakia the cut-off age is fifty-two, while it is fifty-five in Cyprus. In Ukraine, Russia, Poland, and Turkey there is no upper age limit for IVF. For this reason, fertility clinics in these countries are popular destinations for "fertility tourism."

Another hurdle is health. Before having IVF, the causes of infertility, like endometriosis or uterine fibroids, must be diagnosed and treated to increase the chances of success. Of course, the treatment itself can also sidestep some problems, such as blocked fallopian tubes, because the procedure bypasses tubal damage by transferring embryos directly into the uterus. Underlying health conditions—for example, thyroid dysfunction—can also impair fertility and must be addressed. Older patients are sometimes expected to go through an additional screening process to ensure that their general health is sufficient to undergo treatment. They might be required to have an EKG and a cardiac stress test before they are given clearance to have IVF, because pregnancy stresses the heart and circulatory system, especially for older patients. Some patients are considered to be "poor prognosis" candidates for IVF because of their low AMH, high FSH, or "advanced age." These patients may be discouraged from having IVF or actively refused the procedure because it is deemed a "futile" treatment for them.

IVF success rates can be lower in overweight and obese women too, so some patients are denied fertility treatments because they are deemed "too fat." The bar can be high to get access to IVF. The "best candidates" are those who possibly need it less: people who are young and healthy, and who have more eggs. Many patients are also expected to undergo genetic testing or psychological counseling, or to fulfill other requirements before they can get help. While it is understandable that doctors want to ensure that their patients are medically fit to carry a baby and that the treatment wouldn't be pointless, it seems unfair that infertile women have to jump through so many hoops. Although there is no "license" for becoming parents in the usual way, there is a loss of liberty and agency for people with infertility who have to ask permission for just a chance to get pregnant, while the decision-making is left in the hands of others. Couples who try to conceive naturally are not held up to such scrutiny or vetted for their suitability to have kids, no matter what their state of finances, health, weight, or age. When a couple is *in flagrante delicto*, it's not as though a doctor in a white lab coat with a clipboard suddenly materializes, demanding proof of their eligibility to try to have children.

On Pins and Needles

I was anxious to start IVF, but there was one advantage to waiting three months before having the procedure. This three-month window of preconception is the time frame for eggs to mature before ovulation, so it was the perfect opportunity for me to improve my egg quality through nutrition and supplements. One of the first things any fertility clinic will do is advise you to take a prenatal vitamin to prepare for a healthy pregnancy. This ensures that the body is getting adequate amounts of vitamins, including B vitamins, especially folic acid to prevent major birth defects of the baby's brain and spine; antioxidants; and vitamin D, as well as minerals such as magnesium, iron, zinc, and calcium. One of the best ways to obtain these nutrients is through food, so it is recommended that people about to undergo IVF have a diet rich in fruit and vegetables, whole grains, healthy fats, lean meat, nuts, beans, and legumes. Some clinics suggest avoiding sugar, processed or fried foods, and alcohol, because they can damage mitochondria (which function like batteries for our cells), causing premature aging of the egg cells. Of course, smoking should be avoided, as well as illicit drugs. As a coffee lover, I was disappointed to learn that recent studies suggest caffeine can decrease the success rate of IVF. There are so many "dont's" when it comes to trying to conceive. While there are some things that definitely pose a risk to women who are trying to get pregnant, they also become targets of the morality police and unfairly judged for their diets and habits. I asked Dr. Ross if I should avoid sugar carbs, tea, and coffee during this time. Ever sensible and practical, she replied, "Everything is fine in moderation."

As we've seen already, many popular herbal supplements are at best worthless, but at worst dangerous for women who are pregnant or trying to conceive. On the other hand, certain supplements are recommended by some fertility clinics to enhance egg health, especially for patients with diminished ovarian reserve. Omega-3 fatty acids are thought to help produce higher-quality eggs and improve reproductive functioning in advanced maternal age. Coenzyme Q10 (CoQ10) is a nutrient believed to boost mitochondrial function and improve the quality of eggs. Melatonin is a hormone that has antioxidant qualities and is believed to encourage ovarian function and scavenge the free radicals that can damage sperm and egg DNA. The amino acids L-carnitine and L-arginine improve sperm health and are also said to improve quality and quantity of eggs. Myo-inositol is a sugar made in the body that is believed to produce better-quality embryos, and is used primarily for women with PCOS to normalize menstrual cycles.

Dehydroepiandrosterone (DHEA) is a naturally occurring hormone that is thought to boost egg quality and improve pregnancy rates in women who are "poor responders" to IVF stimulation medication. Pyrroloquinoline quinone (PQQ) is a vitamin-like compound believed to fight mitochondrial damage, which is touted as an anti-aging secret to give eggs the energy they need to grow and divide properly. Early research into the coenzyme NAD+ (nicotinamide adenine dinucleotide) and its precursors (nicotinamide riboside, or NR, and nicotinamide mononucleotide, or NMN) focused on their anti-aging effects, while it is thought that they might help fertility too by improving the quality of "aging" eggs. Resveratrol, a plant compound found in red grapes and red wine that is a popular beauty elixir in skin care products, might be effective at improving egg quality and maturation. Other adjuncts include ovarian rejuvenation, such as the use of ovarian platelet-rich plasma (PRP) injections and human growth hormones (or HGH, proteins produced by the pituitary gland that spur growth in children and adolescents and are believed to slow the aging process), to help with low egg reserves. All of these (often very expensive) supplements show exciting promise for infertility, especially in studies on animals (usually mice, fruit flies, and ringworms), although they are still experimental and there is no firm evidence for their effectiveness in humans.

Many women also experiment with alternative medicine in conjunction with IVF. Dealing with infertility can leave people feeling vulnerable and powerless, because control is given over to doctors and nurses, so alternative therapies can help people feel empowered to take charge of their fertility. Popular integrative modalities include hypnotherapy, aromatherapy, meditation, massage, yoga, and LED light therapy. Some men try out alternative therapies for fertility too. An interesting one that Matt and I encountered was the use of self-hypnosis to increase sperm count, motility, and morphology through visualizing these improvements.

"Imagine your sperm growing in number," was a self-hypnotic suggestion made by a hypnotherapist. "Picture your sperm as healthy, strong, and ready to penetrate that egg."

Just as with the herbal supplements and magical remedies, we need to be careful of outrageous claims about curing infertility. Many books and costly programs and apps are available that promise to help you get pregnant within a single cycle or two. But as the saying goes, if it sounds too good to be true, then it probably is. Overall, the evidence for the efficacy of complementary therapies is still slim, but some of the more innocuous ones may be worth trying anyway for self-focus and relaxation. If they help people to relax, then that is no small feat.

IVF is stressful—there's no doubt about that. Patients have rated the stress of IVF as more stressful than, or as stressful as, any other major life event, including divorce or the death of a family member. The anxiety comes from the side effects of medication, financial worries, and the uncertain outcomes of the treatment. Many patients fret that this stress can affect their chances of success with IVF. As we know, there's nothing more stressful than being told to *not* be stressed. Fortunately, studies show that physiological and psychological stress do not negatively affect IVF outcomes. (Some research even suggests that high cortisol concentrations, which correlate with stress, may have positive effects on pregnancy rates.) But there are ways to cope with the stress of IVF. Self-care is important; getting rest, eating a balanced diet, and moderate exercise can be beneficial, as well as giving yourself rewards throughout the process (think: seeing a movie, listening to music, or having a facial). A strong circle of understanding friends and family is invaluable during this time. Alternatively, a therapist, counselor, or support group can offer sympathetic care to ease anxiety. To reduce the stress surrounding IVF, one Israeli study explored the effects of therapeutic laughter. Immediately after transfer, when patients stay lying down to allow for the embryos to settle in, one group received a fifteen-minute visit from a trained "medical clown" who performed a comedy routine. The study found that those who were entertained by the clown were slightly more likely to get pregnant.

Acupuncture has become a popular alternative therapy for patients to manage their IVF anxiety. This is the practice of inserting thin needles into specific points in the skin to relieve health conditions—in this case, infertility. In fact, many fertility clinics recommend the use of acupuncture as a complement to IVF to reduce stress, regulate hormones, and improve ovarian and uterine blood flow, which can improve the chances of implantation. (For this same reason, other clinics like mine suggest taking one baby aspirin per day to improve blood circulation and reduce inflammation.) Practitioners recommend having acupuncture one to two times a week during the ninety days of preconception, and also on the days of embryo retrieval and transfer. This can work out to be rather costly. Some studies show impressive data, suggesting that acupuncture improves pregnancy rates and live births for assisted conception, although the jury is still out on the matter. Anecdotally, many people swear that acupuncture helped them to have success with IVF, but the scientific community puts this down to the placebo effect.

In the spirit of "don't knock it until you try it," I decided to try acupuncture. I saw David, an acupuncturist who specializes in infertility. During these sessions, I lay down on a massage table in a private cubicle, fully clothed. David inserted hair-thin needles into my skin at various points on my body. In some areas I felt a mild stinging sensation, which I was told means "it's working," while in other places I didn't feel anything at all. I had assumed the needles would be placed in my pelvic region, but I was surprised to find they were also used in my feet, chest, ears, and forehead. These points are said to stimulate the reproductive system and improve the flow of energy (or "chi") in the body. When the needles were in place, David dimmed the lights and turned on some soothing New Age music, giving me some quiet time to let the needles do their work. This felt relaxing—that is, except for the time the guy in the next cubicle started snoring.

One day, when my acupuncture session was finished, I went to the front desk to pay the receptionist.

"Um, you have a needle sticking out of your neck," she observed.

I touched my throat and yes, there was a shiny silver needle lodged there. Grossed out, I pulled it out of my skin. Then I patted myself down, and to my horror I discovered that the acupuncturist had accidentally left another needle in my ear and one on the top of my head too. I removed them and handed them over to the receptionist.

"Yuck," she muttered, taking them from me in disgust and tossing them in the trash can.

At this point I decided that acupuncture wasn't for me.

The Eleventh Hour

I'd been told to call the clinic when I started my next period, although I secretly hoped that I wouldn't need to do IVF after all. I'd been lurking on online support forums and had read several anecdotes about women who were ready to start IVF but, ironically, fell pregnant naturally at the last minute. Although I knew my odds of this happening were very low—1 percent, according to my previous doctor—I still hoped for that miraculous pregnancy at the eleventh hour.

But it was not to be for me: my period came right on time. I'd always had a very regular cycle of twenty-six days.

I called the clinic and was told to start taking a birth control pill on the third day of my cycle.

Why would I take the pill when I'm trying to get pregnant? I wondered.

It may seem counterintuitive to take the contraceptive pill when trying to conceive, but there are good reasons for doing so. Taking birth control pills for a few weeks or more before IVF decreases the chances of cysts that could interfere with starting the IVF cycle, and may help the ovaries to respond better to stimulation medication. This also allows the doctor to control the timing of the IVF cycle. Some clinics do something called "Batch IVF," in which the menstrual cycles of multiple women are programmed so they can all undergo the process at the same time. (This is more for the convenience of the clinic than the patient, and can make the process feel less personal and a bit like a factory line.) IVF involves several steps; at the start of my next period, I would have blood work and a baseline ultrasound, and if these were normal, we would then proceed to ovarian stimulation and monitoring, egg retrieval, sperm retrieval, fertilization, and embryo transfer.

Here I was, about to start IVF. I felt anxious and even a little scared, but also grateful for the opportunity to try it. I thought back to the words of my former gynecologist when he barked, "You're not a Hollywood celebrity who can afford expensive infertility treatments."

He was wrong, in that IVF is mainstream nowadays, and many "regular people" like me have the procedure. But it is true that lots of Hollywood stars and celebrities have used IVF to start or complete their families. Michelle Obama and former president Barack Obama suffered a miscarriage that left them feeling "failed" and "broken," so they went on to use IVF to conceive their two daughters. Chef Gordon Ramsey had a low sperm count from standing next to hot stoves for so many years, while his wife Tana faced PCOS. They suffered several miscarriages before going through IVF and becoming parents to four children, two single births and one set of twins. Talk show host Jimmy Fallon and his wife, Nancy, revealed they had an "awful struggle with infertility" for five years before having their two daughters with the help of IVF and surrogacy. Nicole Kidman, Sarah Jessica Parker, and Kim Kardashian also used surrogates to have their babies. (Some celebrities choose to use a "social surrogate," not for medical needs, but for personal ones. This decision is often criticized, that pregnancy doesn't "fit into their schedules," or as vanity, that they don't want to be "disfigured" by pregnancy. But pregnancy can threaten the careers of some women if they either take time out from work or if their body changes.) Brooke Shields, Jennifer Lopez, Tyra Banks, Chrissy Teigen, Mariah Carey, Courteney Cox, and Celine Dion are just a few of the many celebrities who used IVF to conceive their children.

But as we know all too well, IVF doesn't always work. Actress Emma Thompson had her first child with the help of IVF, but then she suffered secondary infertility and was unable to get pregnant again with subsequent rounds, so she adopted her teenage son, a former Rwandan child soldier. Actor Hugh Jackman married Deborra-Lee Furness when he was twenty-seven and she was forty. They fought a long battle with infertility and had multiple failed attempts at IVF before they welcomed their son and daughter through adoption. Many other Hollywood actors have had children well into their late forties and early fifties, although it is speculated they had IVF, and possibly used donor eggs.

"If they're over forty, they're probably using IVF," Dr. Ross confirmed.

This highlights an unfair stigma surrounding the need to use IVF, and an unfounded pride in getting pregnant naturally. But of course, if people in the public eye don't want to discuss their fertility, they have an absolute right to their privacy and don't deserve to be "outed" from the infertility closet by the media. On the other hand, when high-profile people open up about their infertility struggles, it helps the rest of us know there are solutions, and helps us feel like we're not alone.

Back at the clinic I was having my baseline ultrasound. The technician had been chatty, but she suddenly went silent.

This isn't good, I thought.

I suspected something was wrong when she left the room and returned with Dr. Ross in tow.

The doctor frowned as she looked at the screen.

"Yes, I see it," she said under her breath.

"See what?" I asked nervously.

"A cyst."

Ovarian cysts are solid or fluid-filled sacs that form on an ovary. Some cysts are functional, meaning they are a part of the menstrual cycle, and we may often get them without even knowing it. These are different from nonfunctional cysts, such as those that appear as a result of PCOS or those caused by cancer. Functional cysts are harmless and usually disappear on their own within a month or two. My cyst was functional, however, it was a corpus luteum cyst that was producing estrogen, which may interfere with egg development. Most clinics wait for these kinds of cysts to resolve before continuing IVF treatment. However, taking the contraceptive pill was supposed to *prevent* cysts. When dealing with the human body, which is temperamental and unpredictable, there will likely be glitches and setbacks along the way.

"I'm so sorry," said Dr. Ross, "but we'll have to delay your cycle."

Playing God

Dr. Ross switched me to a different birth control pill and increased the dosage to prevent new cysts from forming. (Today's pills contain dramatically lower amounts of hormones than the first marketed pills did.) Then one month later I was back at the clinic for a second baseline ultrasound. I was watching TV in the waiting room when a news report appeared about an IVF mix-up. A woman became pregnant with another couple's child when medical staff transferred the wrong embryos to her uterus. The mistake was only discovered when a nurse called the patient by a different name as she was wheeled out of the operating room. A number of IVF mix-ups have appeared in the news over the years. In another instance, an embryo mix-up at a clinic in Los Angeles meant that two couples gave birth to each other's babies and unwittingly raised the other parents' child for nearly three months before learning the truth. I fell down a rabbit hole, reading horrifying stories of eggs and embryos that were lost in storage errors or destroyed in accidents. Some examples of IVF negligence weren't accidental, but downright malpractice. In several cases of "serial sperm donors," unethical doctors have used their own sperm to fertilize the eggs of women who seek an anonymous donor when undergoing IVF.

In a famous story of gross negligence, Natalie Denise Suleman became a tabloid sensation in 2009 when she gave birth to a set of octuplets, the media dubbing her "Octomom." She had already conceived six children via IVF when she requested to have her remaining frozen embryos transferred into her uterus so they would not be destroyed. It was later discovered that her fertility doctor, Dr. Michael Kamrava, had transferred *twelve* embryos all at once. His reason for doing so was patient autonomy. He argued, "The ultimate decision should be largely driven by the patient's wishes." Another patient of his, a forty-eight-year-old, suffered complications when she became pregnant with quintuplets after receiving seven embryos. The doctor's medical license was later revoked. A decade before these cases there was an original "Octomom" who is lesser known today: Mandy Allwood took powerful fertility drugs and discovered she was expecting octuplets, but tragically, at twenty-four weeks she miscarried all eight babies, one by one, over three days. After her loss, she suffered phantom pregnancies in which she said she could still feel her babies kicking. These were absolutely *not* the kinds of IVF experiences I wanted to hear of when I was about to start it myself. But Dr. Ross reassured me that out of the millions of IVF cycles performed every year, cases of medical malpractice are extremely rare.

These quirky stories only add to the bad press that IVF has had over the decades. From the days of Gregory Pincus and his fatherless rabbits, in vitro fertilization has raised many ethical concerns. These fears have often been explored in speculative fiction. As mentioned before, *Brave New World* is about a dystopian future in which people's traits and social status are determined before they are born. In a baby-making laboratory called the Hatchery, eggs and sperm are mixed together in glass dishes and grown in an artificial womb, where they can be cultured with nutrients to breed intelligent citizens, or spiked with poisons to create an underclass of subhuman servants. In the science fiction film *The Matrix*, human beings are no longer born but grown in endless fetus fields and then used as a source of power. The movie *Gattaca* is about a grim future society in which potential children are conceived through genetic selection to ensure they possess the best traits of their parents. In a dark side to IVF, Robert Edwards, who we know to be one of its inventors, was an active member of the British Eugenics Society. He once wrote, "Soon it will be a sin of parents to have a child that carries the heavy burden of genetic disease. We are entering a world where we have to consider the quality of our children." People are still fearful of "genetic engineering" and "designer babies" who are bred for preferred traits such as eye color, hair color, athleticism, and height (although choosing such physical and personal qualities is simply part of the process when selecting a match for donor eggs or sperm). Preimplantation genetic screening, which tests for chromosomal normalcy and allows parents to choose the sex of their babies, and polygenic screening for disease risks, are controversial modern tests, although they are becoming commonplace adjuncts to IVF.

Since its inception, IVF has sparked fervent moral debate and controversy. When Louise Brown was born, her parents received death threats and hate mail. In protest, one critic sent them a package containing a broken test tube and a toy fetus covered in fake blood. Some people believe that IVF is unnatural and that children should only be born as part of an intimate physical relationship between a (preferably married) man and woman. In the wholesome folklore of conception, babies are delivered by storks or found in cabbage patches; they aren't made in test tubes in a laboratory. People fear that these "test-tube babies" are somehow alien and unnatural, that they will be born weak or abnormal, and that they will look or act unusual. Even before her mother was able to hold her newborn, Louise had undergone around sixty different tests to ensure she was "normal." But these concerns are unfounded today. Scientific studies show that while there is a small increase in low birth weight and premature birth, IVF babies seem to be just as healthy as those conceived naturally.

IVF faces criticism from some religious quarters too. Religious groups such as the Roman Catholic Church fiercely oppose IVF because they believe that infertility is God's will and to go against it is wrong. Their solution is that infertile couples should adopt children or go into providing foster care instead. According to the Church, using donor eggs or sperm or using a surrogate introduces a third or even a fourth person into a relationship, and some see this as committing adultery. (Negative views against using donors and surrogates can also reflect prejudice against sexual orientation, because LGBTQ people often use these methods of having children.) Some religious leaders have expressed concerns that IVF has turned conception into a trade in human eggs and surrogacy that "cheapens life." They argue that IVF results in millions of surplus embryos being abandoned or left to die. Some equate this with murder, because they believe that from the point of conception, the embryo is a human being to be treated with respect and dignity, rather than as a disposable commodity. Personhood, the status of being a person, is a controversial topic in law and society. In "pro-life" states, an embryo is seen as a "judicial person," an entity with legal rights, although these rights are the subject of much debate. By definition, a human life may be considered a human person at fertilization. There is an individual interpretation to personhood too: from the perspective of some people who undergo IVF, their hard-earned embryos *are* their babies.

Amid all of this squabbling, couples of faith are the ones who lose out. They are judged by their community for using fertility treatments, but also judged when they don't conceive. When they don't have kids, it is often assumed they are willfully avoiding parenthood. People gossip: *Are they not having children deliberately? Are they using contraception? Having abortions?* As we've already seen, some cruelly say to infertile couples, "God doesn't want you to have children," or "God has other plans for you." It's enough to bring on a crisis of faith for some. Such pronouncements can be hurtful and ignorant, but they are often influenced by church opinion. For example, Pope Francis denounced fertility treatments for treating children as "a right rather than a gift to welcome" and denounced IVF as "playing God." (But perhaps it's playing God to tell other people what to do with their bodies.) On the other hand, when Louise Brown was born, Cardinal Albino Luciani (who was soon to become Pope Paul I) was unexpectedly sympathetic. He refused to criticize her parents, acknowledging that they simply wanted to have a baby.

I simply wanted to have a baby too, and IVF was my only hope at this point.

But my second baseline ultrasound was a repeat of the first one. I had another cyst.

"I'm sorry," said Dr. Ross, "but we'll have to delay your cycle again."

This is never going to work, I thought, as I climbed into my car and cried all the way home.

That night I received a phone call from Dr. Ross.

"Don't worry," she said soothingly. "Things may look rough now, but I'm going to create the perfect protocol for you to give you the best chance at having a baby."

Trust the Process

There are many different kinds of IVF protocols, each with its pros and cons, and fertility doctors choose the type that is best suited to the patient's individual situation. If I hadn't developed cysts, I would've been placed on a short protocol and started "stimming," which is in-group lingo for ovulation stimulation, taking fertility drugs to stimulate the ovaries to produce follicles that might contain eggs. Because I was prone to developing cysts, I was placed on a long protocol. This involves an extra step, down-regulation, taking medication to temporarily shut off the body's process of hormone and egg development.

"This switches off the ovaries," explained Dr. Ross, "so we can switch them back on at the right time. It also prevents cysts from forming."

I was prescribed a drug called Lupron (leuprolide acetate), and was surprised to learn that it has an interesting provenance. Lupron was originally a chemotherapy drug for breast, ovarian, and endometrial cancers, and then it came to be used for endometriosis and uterine fibroids. It is also used to treat early-onset puberty and as part of transgender hormone therapy. Men use Lupron too, to treat the symptoms of prostate cancer. I was astonished to discover that high doses of the drug have been used to chemically castrate pedophiles for sex offender therapy.

As part of my IVF cycle, I had to inject a small dose of the drug into my stomach every morning for three weeks. Then I returned to the clinic for my third baseline ultrasound.

Matt and I held our breath as we watched the murky gray image on the screen.

"You are cyst-free!" exclaimed Dr. Ross.

We were relieved, to say the least. Finally, we were moving forward.

"Sometimes you just have to trust the process," said Matt.

The old sporting slogan "trust the process" became a mantra for my IVF journey, reminding me to let go and have confidence that things would work out in the end.

With a clear baseline ultrasound, I was finally given the green light to start stimming. There are two main types of medication used to stimulate the ovaries: human chorionic gonadotropins (HCG), which contain FSH, and human menopausal gonadotropins (HMG), which contain both FSH and LH. (I was fascinated to learn that early pharmaceutical HCGs were extracted from the urine of pregnant women, while HMGs were extracted from urine taken from postmenopausal nuns.) These gonadotropins are taken in conjunction with an antagonist that prevents the ripe eggs from being released too early. When it comes to infertility treatments, no two protocols are the same. Some patients may be prescribed fewer drugs or more drugs, depending on their situation. I was placed on a regimen of Follistim and Menopur, along with Cetrotide to delay ovulation until my egg retrieval. There are many different brands of fertility medications, although the difference is akin to Coke versus Pepsi. The one thing that IVF medications all have in common is that they are ridiculously expensive, especially in the US, where the market for fertility drugs is worth about $750 million annually. There is obvious sexism in the pharmaceutical industry when it comes to fertility. Viagra and other drugs used to treat erectile dysfunction in men cost only about $30–$70 per pill, while fertility drugs for women run into many thousands of dollars per cycle.

I had been poked and prodded for years, but now it was about to get a lot worse. Unlike the oral tablets I took for my IUIs, but similar to the Lupron injections, gonadotropins are taken as injections each day until the follicles are mature. But I wouldn't be visiting the clinic for daily jabs; we had to do them ourselves. Matt gave the injections to me, to help share the workload.

"I'd take them for you if I could," he said.

It was a thoughtful and sweet sentiment, but despite being six foot four, Matt had a needle phobia and was terrified of having injections, even his annual flu shot.

Prior to starting the shots, Matt and I attended an injection training class with a nurse. It was a steep learning curve. Some medications need to be mixed; for example, Menopur comes as a vial of powder that is reconstituted with a sodium chloride solution before it is injected. The injections are subcutaneous; that is, they are injected just under the skin using a very small needle. They are typically injected into the stomach, where there is plenty of fatty tissue, about one inch away from the belly button. To make the injections easier, I used ice to numb the area and pinched the skin at the injection site. The shots still hurt sometimes, but I tried to stay mindful as I had each one, to remember their purpose and keep my eye on the prize. We were told that to avoid skin irritation, the same spot should not be injected more than once. But after weeks of multiple daily injections, I had become a pincushion, and my belly was covered in red, purple, and yellow bruises.

"Where do you want this injection?" asked Matt one day a couple weeks into the regimen.

"Find an unbruised area," I replied.

But there weren't any.

Once the IVF cycle finally starts, things move pretty fast. The cycle must be monitored regularly to gauge the patient's response to the medications. The clinic becomes a second home, to have ultrasounds to track the growth of the follicles, as well as blood work to measure estrogen levels to see if the dosage of the medication should be modified. Fertility medications are infamous for their intense side effects, which include mood changes, headaches, bloating, and breast tenderness. I felt some irritability and anxiety, along with cramping and nausea. Cruelly, taking fertility medications mimics pregnancy. Some people can have an exaggerated response to the medication and develop a condition called ovarian hyperstimulation syndrome (OHSS) in which the ovaries swell and leak fluid into the body, causing nausea, bloating, and abdominal pain. (It was to avoid this particular condition that the "French fries will get you pregnant" legend arose.) Women at higher risk for OHSS include those who have PCOS or who develop a large number of follicles.

When the cycle has officially begun, an ultrasound is performed for an antral, or "resting," follicle count, to count the number of follicles that are developing in the ovaries. On the ultrasound screen, these small sacs filled with fluid look like black lumps bulging in the ovaries. They grow at a rate of about 2 mm per day, and are considered mature when they are 16–20 mm in diameter. In some cases, if the ovarian follicle response is poor, meaning there are fewer than three follicles, the cycle may be canceled. IVF cycles might be canceled if the doctor feels the cycle is not optimal for the best outcome. The IVF process is full of perils and pitfalls, and might end abruptly at any point along the way. Fortunately, I wasn't at risk of having my cycle canceled, although I had only ten follicles, while some other women have fifteen to twenty of them.

"You're just a poor responder," remarked the technician.

It was a discouraging thing to hear. (I would later learn that the long protocol may lead to ovarian over-suppression, resulting in fewer follicles.)

"But it only takes one egg," comforted Dr. Ross when she called me later that night. "And I have good news," she said. "You'll take your trigger shot tomorrow at 9 p.m. sharp."

This was to be my final injection, a shot of the pregnancy hormone HCG, which triggers ovulation. Clinics schedule the shot to be given precisely thirty-six hours before the retrieval, when the eggs are released from the follicles for collection. As a reminder that nothing was going to be easy on this journey, the trigger shot was an intramuscular injection given in the upper outer quadrant of the buttocks.

"Ow!" I hollered as Matt jabbed me with the long, thick needle.

But it's fun trying to get pregnant, isn't it? These words that many had said to me by now came flooding back to taunt me.

No. Trying to conceive *isn't* fun for people with infertility.

All the effort, expense, and pain of infertility and its treatments can leave you feeling bitter toward those who get pregnant by simply having sex.

But now it was show time.

The Retrieval

"I'll be there when you wake up," promised Matt as he gave me a farewell kiss.

It was two days later, and we were at the hospital early in the morning for my egg retrieval. While I was taken to a pre-op holding room to prepare for my procedure, an embryologist ushered Matt to a collection room to provide a semen specimen for the in vitro fertilization.

"Here's the honeymoon suite!" joked the embryologist.

There was the customary plastic-covered couch and specimen cup on the table. Having done this before for both semen analyses and IUIs, Matt was now familiar with the process and less embarrassed than he once was. He knew that the staff don't think twice about it and that the clinic is a no-judgment zone. Their focus is to help their patients achieve pregnancy.

While IVF is emotionally hard on a couple, it is undeniably harder on the woman's body physically. She has to take harsh hormonal medications and undergo numerous invasive tests and surgeries, whereas the man simply provides a sample of sperm. But having said that, many men and partners *do* care. I was lucky that Matt was a patient and supportive husband. He'd been there beside me throughout the entire process. This was in stark contrast to a colleague's conception experience; when she expressed that she wanted to have a baby, her husband replied, "You can do whatever you like, as long as *I* don't have to do anything!" Some men won't make a commitment to conception beyond having sex. Even when there is commitment, infertility can and will wreak havoc on relationships. Infertility takes its toll on a marriage because both members are going through it. Some marriages don't survive the strain of infertility. Matt and I had certainly bickered and argued along the way, but ultimately, the experience made us stronger. To get through infertility, a couple needs to face the challenges together.

I was prepped for surgery and taken into the operating room. The egg retrieval is performed under general anesthetic, and there was a whole team of nurses and doctors on hand who introduced themselves. I felt overwhelmed.

"Everything will be okay," promised Dr. Ross. "I'm good at getting eggs."

She held my hand as I went under.

In the early days of IVF, laparoscopic surgery was used to collect the eggs. Nowadays, the egg retrieval is often done through a procedure called transvaginal ultrasound aspiration. The tip of a thin needle is passed through the top wall of the vagina. Then, using a light suction, the doctor aspirates the follicular fluid to collect the eggs from the follicles.

I woke up feeling slightly groggy from the mild sedation. When my blurry eyes cleared, I saw the number "7" was scribbled on the palm of my hand with a blue ballpoint pen. The recovery room nurse saw me looking at it.

"That means we retrieved seven eggs," she explained.

I was in two minds about the outcome. I was ecstatic that I had produced seven eggs—seven precious chances at life. On the other hand, I was a little disappointed that we had *only* retrieved seven eggs from ten follicles. Unfortunately, not all follicles contain eggs. This is because some follicles are small and immature, so they don't have eggs, while others are large and have formed cysts that don't contain eggs either. In a rare condition called empty follicle syndrome, no oocytes are retrieved from mature follicles, possibly due to a low ovarian reserve. Some patients fear that IVF triggers early menopause by taking too many eggs, but this is just a myth. With a regular menstrual cycle, one egg is lost every month, although approximately one thousand others die in the process. IVF simply captures some of those eggs that would otherwise die.

It's difficult to determine how many eggs "should" be collected during an IVF cycle. The number is influenced by the patient's cause of infertility, age, and the protocol type and medications used. Ultimately, it's not the number of eggs that matter, but their quality.

Dr. Ross entered the recovery room.

"Good work!" she exclaimed.

"But I only have seven eggs."

"Seven eggs is wonderful," she said. "Especially since you only have one working ovary. This means that if you had two working ovaries, you would've had double that number, and that's impressive."

This gave me some much-needed perspective on the matter.

After the retrieval, the collected eggs can be frozen for future use. Egg-freezing, or cryptopreservation, helps women to preserve their fertility if they are about to undergo treatment for cancer. It's also an option for those women who plan to have children later on, but want to avoid future infertility. However, the cost is high for this convenience. Companies like Apple, Facebook, and Google offer egg-freezing as a perk for employees, to give them more freedom to pursue family planning according to their own timeline. Critics say the policy sends the wrong message, that work is more important than family, and that women can't have both at the same time. Men can also freeze their sperm for use in their own future treatment. This can be helpful for men who have low sperm counts, as backup in case a fresh sample doesn't contain enough sperm. The procedure is also useful before a vasectomy, in case he changes his mind later on, or following a vasectomy reversal, to capture a healthy sample before problems set in. Of course, sperm can be frozen for donation to someone else's treatment. Posthumous sperm retrieval is a new procedure that involves collecting sperm from the testes of a deceased man, via surgery or electrical stimulation of the prostate gland. Sperm can be collected and used to successfully produce a healthy child for around forty-eight hours after a man's death. Post-mortem sperm donation is being promoted as a choice for men to become posthumous sperm donors, akin to organ donors, because in many countries demand exceeds supply. It's also an option for widows. Ellidy Pullin welcomed a baby girl fifteen months after her late husband, Olympian and world champion snowboarder Alex "Chumpy" Pullin, died in a spear-diving accident. The baby was conceived via IVF using sperm that had been retrieved from Chumpy immediately after his death.

In a fresh IVF cycle, the eggs that were collected are fertilized with sperm to create embryos. An embryologist performs the actual "in vitro fertilization," when the eggs are combined with the washed and prepared sperm from the patient's partner or a donor. Although the media referred to Louise Brown as a "test-tube baby," her conception actually took place in a petri dish. Today, fertiliza-tion can occur naturally by placing the sperm together with an egg in culture media in a laboratory dish, or by using intracytoplasmic sperm injection (ICSI). This technique was developed in the 1980s to treat male infertility, and gets around compromised sperm by injecting a single, healthy sperm directly into the egg. ICSI is widely used in IVF clinics nowadays, and we used it too, because of Matt's semen issues. The day of egg retrieval becomes ovulation day and is counted as Day 0. When the eggs are fertilized overnight, the resultant embryos will develop in an incubator for three to five days. But sadly, not all eggs create embryos.

On the morning of Day 1, I received a call from the embryologist. Only five of my seven eggs had fertilized overnight. You might recall from high school biology class that eggs are fertilized when a single sperm penetrates the layers of the egg to form a new cell, called a zygote. This is the magical point of conception. From there, the fertilized egg divides into a two-celled embryo that continues to duplicate and divide, a process called mitosis, which is known as the cleavage stage. About three to four days after fertilization, the embryo becomes a mass of sixteen cells that resemble a mulberry, which is why it is named a *morula*, the Latin word for "mulberry." By the fifth or sixth day, the fertilized egg is a rapidly dividing ball of hundreds of cells known as a blastocyst, coming from the Greek words for "sprout" and "capsule." Blastocysts are most commonly used in IVF, and it is at this stage that the embryo is transferred to the uterus via a fresh transfer, usually on Day 5, 6 or 7, or frozen for use in a frozen embryo transfer (FET) at a later stage. (Frozen transfers tend to have a slightly higher success rate than fresh ones, especially with "high responders," possibly because the uterus is more receptive after a "rest.") But not all embryos make it to the morula or blastocyst stages.

On Day 2, Dr. Ross called and told me only four of the five embryos had survived the night. The fifth embryo had "arrested," meaning it had stopped growing. This numbers game is known as IVF attrition, which is the rate at which viable embryos taper off once they are in the lab and growing. (In some clinics, embryos are only checked for fertilization and then again on the day of the transfer, because they are sensitive to light and temperature changes, and checking them daily can stress the embryo and disrupt development.) This result meant there would be no biopsy for genetic testing, because PGS is usually done with five or more embryos. I was devastated at the loss of my would-be babies. It was a reminder that there are no guarantees with IVF and that it can fail at any point. Sometimes, when there is attrition in embryo growth and the developmental potential of the eggs is unknown, a Day 3 transfer will be done with fresh embryos, because the uterine environment may actually encourage cell growth, making it more likely that the embryos will reach the blastocyst stage and implant into the uterine wall.

"We're going to do a Day 3 transfer," Dr. Ross announced. "The womb is always better than any lab."

The Transfer

The next day we went back to the hospital for our transfer. We were excited because Matt was allowed to attend the procedure. We were told not to wear perfumes or scented deodorant, makeup, or hair products, because odors can be toxic to the fragile embryos. But when we arrived, there was more bad news in store for us; only three of the four embryos had survived. We were terribly sad to hear of the loss of yet another embryo. With the drop-off rate, we'd gone down from ten follicles to seven eggs to just three embryos.

Then Dr. Ross had some surprising news for us.

"We're going to transfer all of them at once," she said.

All of them?

Most clinics will transfer only one or two embryos at a time. Even single embryos can split after transfer, resulting in multiples. Based on the woman's age, three might be transferred, but no more, to avoid another Octomom. I had recently turned thirty-seven, and the clinic team believed that having all three embryos transferred would give me the best chance at having a baby. I was happy that all of my embryos would be given a "chance," but I was also somewhat disappointed. I'd hoped to have one or two leftover embryos to freeze for use in a second attempt if necessary, or at best, a "spare" to try for a second child someday.

Then I panicked at the thought of triplets.

"What are my chances of having triplets?" I asked.

"The odds are very low at about 3 percent," the embryologist reassured me.

Then he handed me a photograph. It was an image of our embryos. They looked like little flowers. There is a complex grading system of embryos at the cleavage stage, rating them for the number of cells that make up the embryo, the amount of fragmentation, and the symmetry of the cells. We were told that we had one high-quality embryo with eight equal cells and no fragmentation, while the other two were rated fair. The lowest rating is poor. However, these grades are crude predictors for pregnancy chances.

"Even though an embryo looks good, it doesn't mean that it *is* good," he explained. "And even if an embryo looks bad, it doesn't mean that it *is* bad."

They looked perfect to me.

I hoped we were looking at our very first baby photo.

A "transfer" refers to the transferal of an embryo or embryos into the uterus. Some clinics perform a mock embryo transfer prior to the real one as a "trial run" to allow the doctor to determine the best route and the ideal location to place the embryo in the uterus. The media tends to incorrectly call the transfer "implanting," but technically, that refers to the next stage, implantation, if and when the embryo attaches to the lining of the uterus. This marks the beginning of pregnancy. Unfortunately, a doctor can't actually *implant* the embryo. If only they could. But to try to aid in implantation, many IVF "add-ons" are available that purport to increase the odds of success. These include assisted hatching, in which the embryo is helped to "hatch" from its "shell" by creating a small crack in the zona pellucida, the thick coat that surrounds the embryo. Some clinics use embryo glue, which is not actual glue but a chemical called hyaluronan that is added to the lab dish to increase the chance of implantation. Endometrial scratching involves slightly wounding the uterus to facilitate embryo implantation after IVF. Unfortunately, most of these expensive supplementary procedures have been shown to have little effect on live birth rates. Reports have shown that the primary drive behind the use of add-on treatments was not to improve outcomes for patients, but to increase the profitability of the clinics that offer them. At worst, there is evidence that some add-ons may actually be counterproductive. A study found that time-lapse systems to monitor embryos had higher miscarriage rates compared to traditional incubation. Then there are the foods that allegedly help with implantation, according to folklore, like pineapple core, pomegranate juice, beets, and Brazil nuts. Many women eat these foods following their transfer, although the jury is still out as to whether these actually help or not.

Yet again, I was lying on a hospital bed with my feet up in the stirrups. Dr. Ross placed a speculum into my vagina. This part of the procedure felt just like an IUI, although the stakes were much higher. The embryologist left the room and returned with the embryos loaded into a small catheter. Dr. Ross took the catheter and placed it through my vagina and into the uterine cavity. Ultrasound imaging was used to guide the placement of the catheter, and we all watched as she gently placed the embryos into my uterus.

"I see them," I whispered.

"So do I," said Matt, with tears in his eyes.

The embryos looked like three tiny stars shining in my womb. Little sparks of life.

I instantly fell in love with them.

Over the coming weeks I would talk to them and sing them lullabies.

A mother's love is there, even before the baby is.

The Two-Week Wait

After the transfer I was sent home armed with instructions to treat myself like I was already pregnant. In the early days of IVF, women were placed on strict bed rest for two weeks after an embryo transfer. This is no longer recommended, because inactivity can lead to blood clots and affect circulation, which isn't good for the uterus. Most doctors will suggest taking it easy for a day or two, avoiding strenuous activity or vigorous exercising, before carrying on with daily life as normal, including going to work, doing gentle exercise, or traveling if needed. During these two weeks, known as the luteal phase of the cycle, I was told to pamper myself, get plenty of sleep, eat a healthy diet, and keep taking my medications. As part of this presumptive pregnancy, there was even more medication. Since the retrieval, I was already taking progesterone supplements to help prepare the lining of the uterus to be ready to receive and nourish the embryos. I was also wearing estrogen patches on my stomach, to allow the hormone to be absorbed through the skin, to help thicken the lining of my uterus. That night, when I inserted the progesterone vaginal gel, I couldn't help but think of those women of the past who, in their hopes of getting pregnant, used vaginal suppositories made from mouse mixed with myrrh, or the powdered right testicle of a weasel. I felt very fortunate to be living in an age of modern science.

I would continue to take these medications for the next two weeks before returning to the clinic to have my pregnancy test. This time is an unbelievably stressful and lonely one. I had gone from almost daily care and contact with the clinic to suddenly feeling alone and isolated. It was all up to me at this point. During my two-week wait (or the TWW, as it's known in the community), I turned to the global online community of others who are trying to conceive (TTC). As is the custom with infertility, there were more abbreviations to learn. In this lingo, AF is not what you might think, but refers to "Aunt Flo," the menstrual cycle, while "Baby Dance," or BD, is a euphemism for having sex with the intention of getting pregnant. Whether you are trying to get pregnant naturally or via assisted reproductive technologies, online forums are spaces where people support and encourage each other and share knowledge and personal experience. These groups form a caring network, sending "sticky thoughts" in the hopes that their embryos will implant and "stick" to the uterine lining, and offering "baby dust" to wish someone good luck in getting pregnant. I had lurked on these forums on and off for years, but during my two-week wait they were a godsend.

On Day 6, I had to travel to Las Vegas to attend a conference. Dr. Ross has assured me that it was safe to travel, although it felt absurd to be going to "Sin City" at this time. While colleagues of mine were getting drunk at nightclubs and pigging out at all-you-can-eat buffets, I was popping prenatal vitamins and retiring early to my hotel room to give myself a vaginal suppository. At breakfast the next morning, I had a metallic taste in my mouth. At first, I blamed the buffet omelet, but then it suddenly occurred to me that this might be a pregnancy symptom. I went straight to the forums in search of symptoms of pregnancy, because many people who are trying to conceive engage in a pastime known as "symptom spotting." (Some indulge in wishful thinking and seem to think that anything and everything is a sign of pregnancy.) They report a wide range of symptoms, including nausea, fatigue, food cravings or aversions, tender breasts, and the classic sign, a missed period, but for me it was still too early for the latter. I dug further and read that having a metallic taste in the mouth is indeed a symptom of pregnancy! This is called dysgeusia and is caused by a surge of hormones in the body, especially estrogen. One woman described it as "having a mouthful of loose change or sucking on a handrail." I was cautiously optimistic, but having felt similarly optimistic with my IUIs, only to be let down, I just tried to carry on with my day.

That night at dinner I felt a strange "zap," an electric shock–like sensation on the left side of my pelvis. Minutes later, I felt another "zing" of electricity. These sensations continued throughout the night.

Is this implantation? I wondered.

It was now Day 7, and implantation can occur anytime between Days 6 and 12 after ovulation, or in the case of IVF, after egg retrieval. As we know, implantation is when the embryo adheres to the wall of the uterus. Many women experience signs of implantation when the blastocyst burrows into the lining of the uterus.

Implantation bleeding is light bleeding or spotting, often with a pinkish or brownish discharge, which some mistake as their period. Implantation cramps are similar to menstrual pains that can feel like dull and aching cramps or twinges. Some feel a pulling, prickling, or tingling sensation that is often isolated to one side of the body.

I was pretty sure that what I was feeling were implantation cramps, but I tried to not get too excited just yet.

I returned home to Denver, and over the coming days I devoured the forums, which were addictive to read. I read numerous IVF success stories that gave me reassurance and optimism. People shared their BFPs ("big fat pregnancies")—their positive results on a pregnancy test; sadly, others shared their BFNs ("big fat nothings")—their negative pregnancy tests. The forums are also a place of consolation for IVF failure and pregnancy or infant loss. I was torn up, reading of people's "angel babies," their babies lost to miscarriage, stillbirth, or infant death. I learned that wishing "baby dust" for someone can be triggering for those who have suffered miscarriages or who have birthed stillborn babies. Then I felt a sense of hope at the stories of "rainbow babies," the babies born after losing a pregnancy or child. As I read these personal accounts of infertility, I was struck by the randomness and chaos of conception. There is so much we know about conception, yet still so much we don't know. Medical interventions can help, but doctors don't know everything. When it comes to fertility treatments, we'll never know exactly why something worked or didn't work.

I didn't know these people on the forums personally—they were anonymous—but I truly empathized with their experiences. I was overjoyed by their successes and inspired by them. I was also crushed by the failures some experienced that left me feeling discouraged and depressed.

Then Matt reminded me, "Their infertility is not your infertility."

A Little Bit Pregnant

There's a saying that "you can't be a little bit pregnant." You either *are* pregnant or you're *not*. But I was in a unique situation, where I truly *was* a little bit pregnant. I'd had embryos transferred into my uterus and was told to treat myself like I was pregnant. Moreover, I was *feeling* a little bit pregnant. It was now Day 10 and I had developed more symptoms over the past few days; I was feeling fatigue, bloating, breast tenderness, and mild cramping.

By Day 11, I felt an inexplicable sense of "knowing" that I was pregnant.

But what do I know anyway? I asked myself.

I'd never been pregnant before, I'd never even had a pregnancy "scare," so I honestly didn't know what to expect. Frustratingly, many pregnancy symptoms are also similar to premenstrual syndrome. But it was still too early to have a missed period. It was also too early to have my beta pregnancy test at the fertility clinic. I was very tempted to "cheat" by peeing on a stick, but that merry-go-round had added extra stress during my IUIs. The fertility nurse at the clinic had also advised me against doing this, because taking a test too early can lead to inaccurate results. But I'd always imagined that finding out I was pregnant, or not pregnant, would be an intimate moment that didn't involve a phone call from a nurse.

By Day 13 I simply couldn't wait any longer. I decided to take a home pregnancy test. Conveniently, I still had one left over from the days of my IUIs.

Shaking, I took the test, creating a terrible mess as I did so.

Sitting on the closed toilet seat, I stared at the stick, watching intently as the fluid washed across the results window and the first pink line, the control line, emerged. Slowly, a second pink line appeared. It was the first time in my whole life that I'd seen that second line.

It was a BFP!

Or was it?

The nurse's words repeated in my head, that home pregnancy tests can give false results. A positive test can sometimes be a false positive. When testing too early, a home pregnancy test can pick up the "trigger" instead—the shot used to induce ovulation—because it contains HCG, the same substance detected in a pregnancy test. The trigger shot can remain in the system for up to fourteen days. IVF can also lead to a "chemical pregnancy," which is when an early pregnancy loss occurs shortly after implantation. Some women have chemical pregnancies without even realizing they were pregnant, because they occur before an ultrasound can detect a pregnancy. However, this is not too early for a home pregnancy test to detect levels of the pregnancy hormone. Because more women are having IVF and tracking their HCG levels with home pregnancy tests, people are detecting chemical pregnancies they would otherwise miss. Mistakes can be made in interpreting home pregnancy tests too. The indent line can sometimes look similar to a positive pregnancy test. Evaporation lines can also appear in the results window of a pregnancy test as the urine dries, leaving a faint streak that can look like a positive line. To those who are not familiar with them, indent lines and evaporation lines can look like a "squinter," meaning you have to look closely to see them, but they can leave someone thinking they are pregnant when they are not. For all I knew, Aunt Flo could still be right around the corner.

This had been, without a doubt, the longest two weeks of my life.

On Day 14, my period still hadn't arrived. I kept checking for it feverishly throughout the night. Then early that morning, I went to the clinic for my beta pregnancy test. The anxiety that I might not be pregnant was equal to the excitement that I might be pregnant. I was shaking as the nurse drew my blood.

"The doctor will call you this afternoon with the results," she said.

I couldn't concentrate on my work that day. I spent my time staring at my phone, waiting for the call from Dr. Ross.

Late that afternoon, I received the call.

"Hello?"

I could hear my voice cracking.

"Congratulations!" she said. "You're pregnant!"

I started crying.

Then she started crying.

For so many years I'd cried tears of sadness, which had finally turned to tears of joy.

CONCLUSION

Conceiving of Infertility

It had been a long journey, but it was all worthwhile when, eight months and two weeks later, our son was born. He arrived a few weeks early, although his prematurity was planned; I had to give birth via cesarean section because of the myomectomy I'd undergone years before. During fibroid removal surgery, the doctor cuts deep into the uterine wall, which can increase the risk of the uterus rupturing during labor. Our son was born healthy, notwithstanding all of the scaremongering attributed to IVF. His conception and birth were a miracle to us, but also not so miraculous: the process involved a lot of hard work.

The infertility journey is a combination of hard work, hope, confidence, and science, and for some, faith. But even my pregnancy wasn't without the shadow of infertility: I almost had twins. During week eight of pregnancy, I had a routine ultrasound to detect the fetal heartbeat. While the fetus was developing normally, the technician discovered a second gestational sac. It was empty. This is called a blighted ovum, or an anembryonic pregnancy, when a fertilized egg implants in the uterus and forms a sac and placenta, but then stops developing. It is a type of miscarriage that usually happens between weeks 7 and 12 of pregnancy, occurring in around 30 percent of multiple pregnancies. I was worried that this "missed miscarriage" would affect my son's growth. But Dr. Ross told me that it wouldn't; when a developing twin disappears, it is absorbed by the surviving baby and its mother. This gives the appearance of a "vanishing twin." I felt overjoyed for my growing son, but also confused and saddened by the revelation, and I still grieve for the loss of our vanishing twin.

My son was only about six months old when people started asking, "When are you going to give him a brother or a sister?" Or they'd say, "He'll make a great big brother some day!"

After the stork brings a baby, a second child is usually expected. In Hans Christian Andersen's "The Storks," he writes, "All parents want a little baby, and every child wants a little sister or brother."

Well, yes, our son wanted a sibling.

In Western society, the model family is depicted as having not one but two (or more) children. The heteronormative nuclear family consists of father, mother, and two kids, or 2.5 children, as the saying goes. This stereotype goes back to the old statistical average, and therefore supposedly typical, number of children per household in the US (or 2.4 children in the UK). Preferably, the couple will have both a boy *and* a girl, known as a "pigeon pair" for the fact that pigeons lay two eggs at a time, combined with the old folk belief that the hatchlings are a male and a female. Throughout history, having one child was uncommon. Since the 1980s, it has become much more common, but is still judged by many as somehow abnormal and "sad," and the family seen as "incomplete."

I'd gone from being seen as different for not having kids to being different for having "only" one.

"Just one?" people would ask, somewhat patronizingly.

In the world of infertility treatment, a singleton is the goal, but in society, a "single child" is often stigmatized. This social stigma gave rise to the theory of "only child syndrome," that being a singleton harms the child's personality. Compared to children with siblings, singletons are stereotyped as spoiled, selfish, bossy, socially inept, or lonesome; "an only child is a lonely child," they say. But there is no evidence for these claims, while fortunately, such views are on the decline and the narrative is slowly changing. Many people are happy as a "triangle family" of three, because "onlies" can mean a better quality of life, more time, and less stress for the parents, and for the child as well.

Social pressure aside, once we got past the ups and downs of new parenthood, we decided that we *did* want to try for another child. Growing up, I'd always thought I'd have two kids, just like my parents did. Our personal experiences influence our perception of "normal" family size. But then we faced secondary infertility. As mentioned before, this happens when a woman who's had one successful pregnancy cannot conceive or carry a second pregnancy. Secondary infertility is as common as primary infertility; it makes up about 50 percent of all cases. After previously having kids, many women ask: Why can't I get pregnant again? The good news is that you're more likely to have a successful second pregnancy if you've already had one child. Of course, we already knew why we couldn't get pregnant again. The reasons were the same as the first time around, so the apparent solution was the same: IVF. Matt and I tried IVF again, going into the procedure with some degree of confidence, because the first attempt had worked. And the second time around it *did* work, for a little while.

I miscarried at eight weeks.

A positive pregnancy test isn't always the end of fertility struggles. Sadly, some pregnancies end in miscarriage. More than 80 percent of miscarriages occur within the first trimester of pregnancy. There are many reasons a miscarriage happens, although the cause is often not identified. Early pregnancy loss is much more common than most people realize. About 10 to 20 percent of pregnancies end in miscarriage. However, the actual number is probably higher, because many miscarriages occur very early on, like chemical pregnancies, before the pregnancy is even detected. Pregnancy loss is a common part of the infertility journey for many people, but it is often not talked about. Miscarriage is neglected by the medical community too, and there needs to be more focus on its diagnosis and treatment, and more support for those who experience it. Actress Sharon Stone, who has three adopted children, revealed that she suffered an autoimmune disease and endometriosis that prevented her from having biological children and resulted in multiple pregnancy losses. "We, as females don't have a forum to discuss the profundity of this loss," Stone shared on Twitter. "I lost nine children by miscarriage. It is no small thing, physically nor emotionally yet we are made to feel it is something to bear alone and secretly with some kind of sense of failure. Instead of receiving the much needed compassion and empathy and healing which we so need."

Suffering a miscarriage is a tragedy, at any week or stage of pregnancy. It is the death of a loved one. It is the loss of hopes and dreams. The passing is felt keenly when the pregnancy was so hard won. Pregnancy loss is a deeply heartbreaking experience, and the would-be child is never forgotten. Every year, I still remember my baby's would-be birthday.

"You can just try again," we were told.

But sometimes you can't.

There is often little sympathy for people facing infertility, and especially secondary infertility. This is a lose-lose situation for parents who have "just" one child. Either they are stigmatized for having an only child, or they are deemed selfish for undergoing IVF or other treatments when they already have a child (or more). The desire for another child can sometimes be misconstrued by others as being ungrateful for the one you already have.

"Be grateful you have a kid at all," people would say.

A person can be grateful for what they have, but still feel sad at the same time.

Infertility is a chronic disease that can cause sadness, stress, and feelings of hopelessness and worthlessness. It is a life crisis that is ranked as one of the most serious traumas a person can experience, outside of the death of a mother or father. But its treatment can also affect psychological well-being and reduce quality of life. Research has shown that women undergoing fertility treatments have levels of depression and anxiety similar to those with other chronic diseases, such as heart disease, HIV, and cancer. (The metaphors we use for infertility, describing it as a "struggle" or "battle," are the same we use for cancer.) Women who go through IVF and those who experience a failed attempt have an increased risk of suicide. These findings emphasize that infertility is a critical condition that needs to be taken seriously. Unlike other diseases, the scars from infertility are invisible, making it easy for society to ignore. But when the bruises from infertility treatment are gone, the pain doesn't always magically go away. Studies have shown that psychological symptoms associated with infertility and its treatments can persist even *after* a woman conceives. Conception through assisted reproductive technologies may have an increased risk of depression during pregnancy, the postpartum period, and beyond. Post-traumatic stress disorder is also common in people post-infertility. Even with a babe in arms, the turmoil and trauma of infertility and its treatment can be long-lasting.

Infertility treatment is not a one-size-fits-all solution. Whether facing primary infertility or secondary infertility, whatever the cause, there are many alternative paths to parenthood. Infertility brings such a sense of powerlessness and loss of control that it's important to remember that there are options. Aside from conventional IUI and IVF, these treatments can also be done using donor eggs and/or donor sperm. Surrogacy is an option for those who cannot carry a baby themselves, and it enables one or both parents to maintain a biological link to the child. Instead of destroying remaining embryos or using them in research, embryo donation allows unused embryos remaining from an IVF cycle to be donated to another person or couple, to give them the experience of pregnancy and the birth of a child. Beyond fertility treatments, many choose to become foster parents, providing a temporary living situation for kids whose parents cannot care for them, while adoption is a way to provide a permanent family for children who can no longer be brought up by their biological parents. It's important to remember that along the way, you might change your mind about what you want to do. Infertility isn't linear; you don't know how you will feel about a treatment or a solution until you get there. It's helpful to keep an open mind about options.

When I first entertained the idea of having IVF, I was concerned that it was outdated technology. It had been around for decades already. But fortunately, there are new trends and developments with the treatment, including advances with fertility medications and procedures, leading to significantly improved success rates. (Tip: Be informed by statistics, but not discouraged by them. Know that they are only a guide, and they are always changing.) And there are new technologies on the horizon. In recent years, uterine transplant has become a rapidly evolving field. Uterine transplants are for women with uterine factor infertility, who don't have a uterus or who have had their uterus removed. Uterine transplants from a deceased or living donor could allow them to become pregnant (via IVF) to carry and deliver a baby. At the time of this writing, there have been over one hundred uterus transplants globally, and over a dozen babies have been born from donated uteruses.

Reminiscent of J. B. S. Haldane's theories of "ectogenesis" and Aldous Huxley's *Brave New World*, scientists have also created the "Biobag," an artificial womb resembling a plastic bag that has been used to keep lambs alive outside of their mother's wombs. This technology could one day be applied to premature babies and people with infertility. Haldane is also remembered for coining the term *clone* in human biology, but cloning isn't just the stuff of science fiction anymore. In the future, it may be possible for couples to use reproductive cloning to have genetically related children. Nuclear transfer is another experimental technique, which involves taking the nucleus of an immature egg and placing it into a nucleus-free donated egg, allowing women with less-than-ideal eggs to still have babies. For some, infertility can even be avoided in the first place through fertility preservation and the freezing of eggs, embryos, ovarian tissue, testicular tissue, or sperm for future reproduction.

There are many more discoveries yet to be made to treat the myriad of conditions and circumstances that make up infertility.

It's also important to remember that infertility is an individual experience. As Matt often reassured me when I'd hear of other people's stories, both good and bad, "Their infertility is not your infertility." This book is the story of my infertility, which may resonate with you at times, although my infertility is *not* your infertility. Your experiences will undoubtedly be different from mine. But whatever your unique story, it's okay. It's okay to seek help to have children, and it's okay to have multiples as a result of infertility treatment. It's okay to have two or more children, one child, or none at all, for that matter. In the midst of infertility, it feels all-consuming and endless, but there is a light at the end of the tunnel. Infertility *will* have an end. Sometimes fertility treatment ends in success. Sometimes it doesn't. Other times it ends with acceptance that having children is not going to happen, but that a rich and meaningful life is still possible, even if the outcome wasn't what was originally pictured or hoped for.

Country music star Dolly Parton is an inspirational example. Parton had a traumatic childhood experience. She came from a large family, and when she turned nine, her mother announced that the little girl would be the "mama" of the next baby and tasked her with taking care of the newborn. The family welcomed a boy, and Parton was allowed to name the baby, whom she called Larry. Tragically, he died only four days later. Parton was so distraught that she felt like she'd lost a baby of her own. Her song "Jeannie's Afraid of the Dark" is about child loss, and still reminds her of her little brother. Parton had always wanted children of her own with husband Carl Dean. They'd even picked out a name: "If we'd had a girl, she was going to be named Carla," she said. But Parton suffered from endometriosis so severe and painful that it once caused her to collapse on stage during a performance. She underwent a partial hysterectomy and was told she'd never have children. Parton was plunged into deep depression, going through a "dark time" in which she contemplated suicide. She said she would've "given up every-thing else for motherhood." Over the years, she healed, eventually coming to accept her infertility and to embrace it. Today, Parton runs the Imagination Library, a program that promotes the joys of literacy to young children. Most people know Dolly Parton as the "Queen of Country," but my son knows and adores her as "The Book Lady," as do many other children around the world. She once said:

> I couldn't have children. I tried to for years. I've never been pregnant in my life. When I was a girl and fooling around I was scared to death I'd get pregnant, and then when I got married and wanted to have children I couldn't have any. But I don't miss it. I did for a while, but now I realize that I am everybody's mother.

Whatever your story, you can and will survive infertility.

Infertility has always existed, and people have always tried to make sense of it. In the past, it was understood as punishment for sins, a curse, or an evil spell. Childlessness was once believed to be a weakness and a moral failing, or even considered a psycho-logical disorder. We've moved on from these views, for the most part, although infertility is still stigmatized and minimized. It is dismissed as a "woman's problem," while the needs of men with infertility are ignored. And we are still subjected to unhelpful or ignorant sound bites. We're told that we're "too old to have kids," "not meant to have children," or that infertility is "part of God's plan." Sometimes you can't understand infertility until you go through it yourself. In our ongoing search to make sense of infertility, we have often ended up making nonsense of it instead. Science came along to explain the medical reasons for infertility, in many of its different forms, and to offer possible solutions for some of these, some of the time. But there is the medical reality of infertility, and then there is its purpose. I have spent many years trying to make sense of infertility, but the truth is that infertility is senseless. It is random, chaotic, and unfair. Because infertility is senseless, we can only make sense of our own personal experiences and find meaning in our own journeys.

Speaking for myself, infertility has taught me that I am not broken or abnormal. There is nothing "wrong" with me, and I am not to blame for my fertility problems. Facing infertility has enabled me to develop inner strength, resilience, and determination. Along the way I often felt lonely, but I discovered that I was not alone, because others could relate to me. Many people have been in my shoes, and there is strength in numbers. Infertility made me realize that life is precious, although creating life is not a given; it is a privilege. Infertility would forever change me. The experiences of infertility and loss are not neatly contained in the moment, but now affect the way I see the world. Infertility has become a part of my identity, but I don't let it define me. And finally, surviving infertility showed me that, through my own experiences, I could raise awareness about this very important issue, encourage positive change, and also help others.

I finally found meaning in my fertility journey. I hope you find meaning in yours.

ACKNOWLEDGMENTS

With sincere thanks to my agent Max, editor Lisa, and the entire Broadleaf team for seeing the value and importance in this topic and helping to make this book happen. Thanks to my husband Matt for embarking on this journey with me, for his support throughout the writing process, and for allowing me to share all of the intimate and embarrassing details of our story. Thank you to my amazing son Blade for giving me a reason to write this book, and for being my raison d'être. Last but not least, my gratitude goes to all those who have suffered infertility, both past and present. Thank you for your remarkable courage and strength, and your moving stories that I have preserved within these pages.

NOTES

Introduction

"... Paleolithic fertility charm in the hopes of having children." Alan F. Dixson and Barnaby J. Dixson, "Venus Figurines of the European Paleolithic: Symbols of Fertility or Attractiveness?" *Journal of Anthropology* 2011, 569120.

"... ensuring that the family was not left without a child." Ahmet Berkiz Turp et al., "Infertility and Surrogacy First Mentioned on a 4000-Year-Old Assyrian Clay Tablet of Marriage Contract in Turkey," *Gynecological Endocrinology* 34, no. 1 (2018): 25–27.

"... not being able to get pregnant after six months of trying." Renald Blundell, "Causes of Infertility," *International Journal of Molecular Medicine and Advance Sciences* 3, no. 1: 63–65, https://www.um.edu.mt/library/oar/handle/123456789/22304.

"... a combination of both male and female infertility." Brennan D. Peterson, Lisa Gold, and Tal Feingold, "The Experience and Influence of Infertility: Considerations for Couple Counselors," *The Family Journal* 15, no. 3 (2007): 251–257. doi:10.1177/1066480707301365.

"... more than one hundred million individuals suffer from infertility worldwide." Ali Rahbar and Milad Abbasi, "A Brief Clinical Overview of Etiological Factors in Infertility," *Journal of Infertility and Reproductive Biology* 8, no. 1 (2020): 6–8.

"... ten million babies have been born via assisted technologies." P. Henriksson, "Cardiovascular Problems Associated with IVF Therapy," *Journal of Internal Medicine* 289, no. 1 (2021): 2–11.

Chapter 1

"... They had been waiting for years to become grandparents."
Patrick Jackson, "Couple in India Sue Son for Not Giving Them
a Grandchild," *BBC News*, May 13, 2022, https://www.bbc.
com/news/world-asia-india-61424869.

"... Jamie Buchman in an episode of *Mad About You*." Paul Reiser
et al., "The Unplanned Child," directed by Thomas Schlamme,
Mad About You, season 2 (1993), episode 6.

"... influenced by social and cultural factors, not biological ones."
Gary L. Brase, and Sandra L. Brase, "Emotional Regulation of
Fertility Decision Making: What Is the Nature and Structure
of 'Baby fever'?" *Emotion* 12, no. 5 (2012), 1141–1154.

"... Happy the man whose people are many." Leonie J. Archer et
al., eds. *Women in Ancient Societies: An Illusion of the Night*
(Basingstoke, NY: Palgrave Macmillan, 1994).

"... by definition, one who bore children to continue her hus-
band's lineage." Janice P. De-Whyte, *Wom(b)an: A Cultural-
Narrative Reading of the Hebrew Bible Barrenness Narratives*
(Leiden: Brill, 2018).

"... woe the mother of daughters, the widow." Klaus Bruhn, "The
Predicament of Women in Ancient India," accessed July 17,
2022, http://www.klaus-bruhn.de/mediapool/57/575086/
data/Predicament_geerdes.pdf.

"... especially during times of falling birth rates." Virginia
Abernethy and Garrett Hardin, *Population Politics: The Choices
That Shape Our Future* (London: Taylor & Francis, 2018).

"... penalized bachelors and childless couples." William E.
Phipps, *Clerical Celibacy: The Heritage* (New York: Contin-
uum, 2004).

"... the population of Europe during the Middle Ages." Jenifer
Buckley, *Gender, Pregnancy and Power in Eighteenth-Century
Literature: The Maternal Imagination* (n.p.: Springer Interna-
tional, 2017).

"... giving recommendations like, 'If she is ugly, the advice is: do it
in the dark.'" Aristotle, pseud., *Aristotle's Masterpiece*: or,

The Secrets of Generation displayed in all the parts thereof . . . very necessary for all midwives, nurses, and young-married women, 1694 (London: W. B.).

". . . encouraged couples to have five children per family. Lauren E. Forcucci, "Battle for Births: The Fascist Pronatalist Campaign in Italy 1925 to 1938," *Journal of the Society for the Anthropology of Europe*, 10, no. 4 (2010): 4–13.

". . . sterilized to prevent them from producing 'degenerate' children." Denise Lynn, "Anti-Nazism and the Fear of Pronatalism in the American Popular Front," *Radical Americas* 1, no. 1 (2016): 25–33.

". . . people in Western countries are choosing to have fewer children." Ann Buchanan and Anna Rotkirch, eds., *Fertility Rates and Population Decline: No Time for Children?* (Basingstoke, NY: Palgrave Macmillan, 2013).

". . . impose penalties or taxes on those without children." Jonathan V. Last, *What to Expect When No One's Expecting: America's Coming Demographic Disaster* (New York: Encounter, 2014).

". . . to be impregnated and bear children for them." Margaret Atwood, *The Handmaid's Tale* (New York: Anchor, 1998); Bruce Miller, *The Handmaid's Tale* (TV series), MGM, 2017.

"The Amish are among the fastest growing populations in the world." Donald B. Kraybill, *The Riddle of Amish Culture*, rev. ed. (Baltimore: Johns Hopkins University Press, 2003).

". . . Cooper experimented on his pet dog." Sheynkin, "History of Vasectomy," *Urologic Clinics of North America* 36, no. 3 (2009): 285–294.

". . . not before tens of thousands of men were made infertile against their wishes." Sheynkin, "History of Vasectomy."

". . . women shoulder the responsibility for contraception by undergoing tubal ligation." World Contraceptive Patterns. 2013. United Nations. Department of Economic and Social Affairs. https://www.un.org/en/development/desa/population/publications/pdf/family/worldContraceptivePatternsWallChart2013.pdf.

"... could restore general vigor and sexual potency." Randi Hutter Epstein, *Aroused: The History of Hormones and How They Control Just About Everything* (New York: W. W. Norton, 2018).

"... revived [his] creative power." Diana Wyndham, "Versemaking and lovemaking--W. B. Yeats' 'strange second puberty': Norman Haire and the Steinach rejuvenation operation," *Journal of the History of the Behavioral Sciences* 39, no. 1 (2003): 25–50.

"... an accidental vasectomy that occurred during a hernia operation." Howard H. Kim and Marc Goldstein, "History of Vasectomy Reversal," *Urologic Clinics of North America* 36, no. 3 (2009): 359–373.

"...Women are born with all the eggs they'll ever have... sperm might also be released during wet dreams." Christopher J. De Jonge and Christopher L. R. Barrat, eds., *The Sperm Cell: Production, Maturation, Fertilization, Regeneration*, 2nd ed. (Cambridge, UK: Cambridge University Press, 2017).

"... if it's been over ten years since the vasectomy." A. P. Patel and R. P. Smith, "Vasectomy Reversal: A Clinical Update," *Asian Journal of Andrology* 18, no. 3 (2016): 365–371.

"... barrenness is a common theme in the Bible." Candida R. Moss and Joel S. Baden, *Reconceiving Infertility: Biblical Perspectives on Procreation and Childlessness* (Princeton: Princeton University Press, 2015).

"... as *la ālittu*, 'a woman who does not bear.'" Marten Stol, *Birth in Babylonia and the Bible: Its Mediterranean Setting*, tr. F. A. M. Wiggermann (Netherlands: Brill, 2021).

"... later gave birth to twins." Stephen Brogan, *The Royal Touch in Early Modern England: Politics, Medicine and Sin* (Woodbridge, Suffolk, UK: Boydell & Brewer, 2015).

Chapter 2

"... who witness the birds' nesting behavior and associate them with parenting and fertility." Rachel Warren Chadd and

Marianne Taylor, *Birds: Myth, Lore and Legend* (London: Bloomsbury, 2016).

"The sun is out, birds are singing. The bees are trying to have sex with them, as is my understanding." Matt Groening et al., "Homer vs. Patty and Selma," directed by Mark Kirkland, *The Simpsons*, season 6 (1989), episode 17.

"There would need to be a guy sitting between you and the toilet seat, but yes, absolutely." David Shore and Peter Blake, "Joy to the World," directed by David Straiton, *House*, season 5 (2008), episode 11.

". . . a man only needs to 'stick it inside her and pee.'" Trey Parker, Matt Stone, and Brian Graden, "Miss Teacher Bangs a Boy," *South Park*, season 10 (2006), episode 10.

". . . sex education video *Where Did I Come From?*" Peter Mayle and Arthur Robins, *Where Did I Come From?* (video), starring Howie Mandel Vega 7 Entertainment, 1985.

". . . healthy and safe sex life in the future." Society for Adolescent Health and Medicine, "Abstinence-Only-Until-Marriage Policies and Programs: An Updated Position Paper of the Society for Adolescent Health and Medicine," *Journal of Adolescent Health* 61, no. 3 (2017): 400–403.

". . . 'It's not nice and you'll just have to put up with it.'" Roy Porter and Lesley Hall, *The Facts of Life: The Creation of Sexual Knowledge in Britain, 1650–1950* (New Haven: Yale University Press, 1995).

". . . programs are woefully ineffective." James McGrath, "Abstinence-Only Adolescent Education: Ineffective, Unpopular, and Unconstitutional," *University of San Francisco Law Review* 38 (2004): 665–700.

". . . give up her baby for adoption." Madonna, vocalist, "Papa Don't Preach," by Brian Elliot and Madonna, track 1 on *True Blue*, Sire - Warner Bros, 1986.

". . . unmarked grave in the churchyard." Serena Clark, "Forgive Us Our Trespasses: Mother and Baby Homes in Ireland," *Visual Communication* 20, no. 1 (2021): 124–133.

"... could lead to the birth of a deformed baby." Katherine Harvey, *The Fires of Lust: Sex in the Middle Ages* (London: Reaktion, 2021).

"... explain the mysteries of conception." Sharon N. Covington and Linda H. Burns, *Infertility Counseling: A Comprehensive Handbook for Clinicians* (Cambridge, UK: Cambridge University Press, 2006).

"... the uterus a scrotum, and the labia a foreskin." Thomas Laqueur, *Making Sex: Body and Gender from the Greeks to Freud* (Cambridge, MA: Harvard University Press, 1992).

"... a woman was just a 'deformed male.'" Aristotle, Immanuel Bekker, W. E. Bolland, and Andrew Lang, *Aristotle's Politics: Books I. III. IV. (VII.)* (London: Longmans, Green, 1877).

"... human corpses and animal carcasses to sketch his findings." Peter M. Dunn, "Leonardo Da Vinci (1452–1519) and Reproductive Anatomy," *Archives of Disease in Childhood: Fetal and Neonatal Edition* 77, no. 3 (1997): F249–251.

"... although at the time, he didn't understand what they did." M. M. Mortazavi, N. Adeeb, and B. Latif, et al., "Gabriele Fallopio (1523–1562) and His Contributions to the Development of Medicine and Anatomy. *Child's Nervous System* 29 (2013): 877–880, https://doi.org/10.1007/s00381-012-1921-7.

"... but he confused the follicles with the egg." M. Thiery, "Reinier De Graaf (1641–1673) and the Graafian Follicle," *Gynecological Surgery* 6, no. 2 (2009): 189–191, https://doi.org/10.1007/s10397-009-0466-6.

"... observed sperm with the newly invented microscope." Gayle Davis and Tracey Loughran, eds., *The Palgrave Handbook of Infertility in History* (London: Palgrave Macmillan, 2017).

"... united with 'soil' (menstrual blood) to form an egg." R. V. Short, "Where Do Babies Come From?" *Nature* 403, no. 6771 (2000): 705.

"... with pregnant women so their fertility rubs off." Rosalind Franklin, *Baby Lore: Superstitions and Old Wives Tales from the World Over Related to Pregnancy, Birth and Babycare* (West Sussex, UK: Diggory, 2005).

"... to synchronize with the tides." Amy L. Harris, and Virginia J. Vitzthum, "Darwin's Legacy: An Evolutionary View of Women's Reproductive and Sexual Functioning," *Journal of Sex Research* 50, no. 3–4 (2013): 207–246.

"... more flirtatious, signaling their high-fertility days." Martie G. Haselton and Kelly Gildersleeve, "Human Ovulation Cues," *Current Opinion in Psychology* 7 (2016): 120–125.

"... believing this will 'increase the chances of conception.'" Joel and Ethan Coen, *The Big Lebowski*, Working Title Films, 1998.

"... will be well on their way." Jen Gunter, *The Vagina Bible: The Vulva and the Vagina—Separating the Myth from the Medicine* (New York: Citadel, 2019).

"... 25 percent of the time." Elisabeth Anne Lloyd, *The Case of the Female Orgasm: Bias in the Science of Evolution* (Cambridge, MA: Harvard University Press, 2006).

"... or where you do it either." Judy Barratt, *The Pregnancy Encyclopedia: All Your Questions Answered* (London: Dorling Kindersley, 2016).

"... adoption was recommended as the 'cure.'" Shurlee Swain, "The Interplay between Infertility and Adoption in Policy and Practice in Twentieth-Century Australia," in Gayle Davis and Tracey Loughran, eds., *The Palgrave Handbook of Infertility in History: Approaches, Contexts, and Perspectives* (London: Palgrave Macmillan, 2017).

"Binge drinking, or drinking to excess, can affect people's fertility." Kristin Van Heertum and Brooke Rossi, "Alcohol and Fertility: How Much Is Too Much?" *Fertility Research and Practice* 3 (2017), art. no. 10.

"... opportunity for conception during that cycle closes." Jani R. Jensen and Elizabeth A. Stewart, *Mayo Clinic Guide to Fertility and Conception* (n.p.: RosettaBooks, 2018).

"Monty Python song 'Every Sperm Is Sacred.'" Graham Chapman et al., *Monty Python's The Meaning of Life*, directed by Terry Jones, produced by John Goldstone, Celandine Films, 1983.

"... only 1–2 percent for women who are forty-three or over." Alex Mlynek, "What Are Your Odds of Getting Pregnant Each Month?" *Today's Parent*, May 22, 2018.

"... 38 percent chance of conceiving in just one cycle." Marlies Manders et al., 2015. "Timed Intercourse for Couples Trying to Conceive," *Cochrane Database of Systematic Reviews* no. 3 (2015): CD011345.

Chapter 3

"... for sperm to appear in the semen after a reversal." "Vasectomy Reversal," Mayo Clinic, accessed July 14, 2022, https://www.mayoclinic.org/tests-procedures/vasectomy-reversal/about/pac-20384537.

"... about 15 percent of male infertility overall." Matthew Wosnitzer, Marc Goldstein, and Matthew P. Hardy, "Review of Azoospermia," *Spermatogenesis* 4, no. 1 (2014): e28218.

"... 'Well, it's not *my* sperm count!' she snaps back at him." Mike Judge and Etan Cohen, *Idiocracy*, directed by Mike Judge, Ternion, 20th Century Fox, 2006.

"... who was described as 'fair, good, but barren.'" Paul Chrystal, *When in Rome: Social Life in Ancient Rome* (Oxford, UK: Fonthill, 2017).

"After only one year of marriage, the emperor Caligula ... Pandateria, before having her executed." Mary Taliaferro Boatwright, *Imperial Women of Rome: Power, Gender, Context* (New York: Oxford University Press, 2021).

"Medical documents reported that Henry II of France.... and the couple went on to have ten children." J. Gordetsky, R. Rabinowitz, and J. O'Brien, "The 'infertility' of Catherine de Medici and Its Influence on 16th Century France," *The Canadian Journal of Urology* 16, no. 2 (2009): 4584–4588.

"... No son of mine succeeding." William Shakespeare, *Macbeth*, Side by Sides (Cheswold, DE: Prestwick, 2003).

". . . he determined he was 'unable to have children by her.'" David Starkey, *Six Wives: The Queens of Henry VIII*, reprint ed. (New York: HarperCollins, 2009).

". . . poor nutrition, diabetes, obesity, and sexually transmitted disease." Valerie Shrimplin and Channa N. Jayasena, "Was Henry VIII Infertile? Miscarriages and Male Infertility in Tudor England," *Journal of Interdisciplinary History* 52, no. 2 (2021): 155–176.

". . . accused by many people of having unsuitable seed." Catherine Rider, "Men's Responses to Infertility in Late Medieval England," in Davis and Loughram, *Palgrave Handbook of Infertility*, 273–290.

". . . semen that was 'too hot, too cold, thinne, waterie and feeble.'" Philip Barrough, *The Methode of Phisicke: The methode of phisicke conteyning the causes, signes, and cures of invvard diseases in mans body from the head to the foote. VVhereunto is added, the forme and rule of making remedies and medicines, which our phisitians commonly vse at this day, with the proportion, quantitie, & names of ech [sic] medicine* (London: Printed by Thomas Vautroullier dwelling in the Blacke-friars by Lud-gate, 1583).

". . . and the Woman in the act feeleth his Seed cold, be sure the man is unfruitfull." John Tanner, 1659. *The Hidden Treasures of the Art of Physick* (London: Printed for George Sawbridge, at the sign of the Bible on Lud-gate-Hill, 1659), 346.

". . . hard, red and hot, and fit for the action." Felix Platter, *A Golden Practice of Physick: in five books, and three tomes: after a new, easie, and plain method of knowing, foretelling, preventing, and curing all diseases incident to the body of man: full of proper observations and remedies, both of ancient and modern physitians: being the fruits of one and thirty years travel, and fifty years practice of physick* (London: Printed by Peter Cole, 1662).

". . . lay by his wife 'like a stone in the Wall,' providing her with no sexual satisfaction." Anonymous, *The Un-equal Match: Or, The Old Feeble Taylor's Insufficiency* (London: 1689).

"... suggesting that male clergy 'cured' barren members of their congregation by sleeping with them." Daphna Oren-Magidor, *Infertility in Early Modern England*, Early Modern History: Society and Culture (London: Palgrave Macmillan, 2017).

"... on individuals and their partners can be significant." Ziyan Sheng, "Psychological Consequences of Erectile Dysfunction," *Trends in Urology and Men's Health* 12, no. 6 (2021): 19–22.

"... hormonal imbalances, disease, genetic issues, or infertility." Hagai Levine et al., "Temporal Trends in Sperm Count: A Systematic Review and Meta-regression Analysis," *Human Reproduction Update* 23, no. 6 (2017): 646–659.

"... if they sprouted quickly, this indicated pregnancy." E. Henriksen, "Pregnancy Tests of the Past and the Present," *Western Journal of Surgery, Obstetrics and Gynecology* 49 (1941): 567–575.

"... which proves difficult and embarrassing." Paul Reiser et al., "The Sample," directed by David Steinberg, *Mad About You*, season 4 (1996), episode 18.

"... advertised in long-winded handbills and newspaper advertisements." Jennifer Evans, "'They Are Called Imperfect men': Male Infertility and Sexual Health in Early Modern England," *Social History of Medicine* 29, no. 2 (2016), 311–332.

"... whether it had been caused by venereal disease or subsequent treatment." *British Journal*, 1722, London, England, October 24, 1724.

"... indebted to this Great Medicine for their Heirs." *Daily Journal*, London, England, February 15, 1737, issue 5922.

"... or wearing a special corset designed to prohibit the activity." Anonymous, *Onania; or, The Heinous Sin of Self-Pollution, and All of Its Frightful Consequences, in Both Sexes* (London, 1724).

"... homemade remedies known as 'kitchen physic.'" Leah Astbury, "Fertility in the Early Modern Household," *The Recipes Project: Food, Magic, Art, Science, and Medicine*, May 2, 2019, https://recipes.hypotheses.org/14650#_edn8.

"... shee shall conceaue." Jane Jackson, *Her Booke* (1642), Wellcome Collection, MS373 fol. 82v.

"... furtively sprinkled 'upon the parties meat.'" Sarah Jinner, *An Almanack and Prognostication for the Year of Our Lord 1659* (London: 1659), sig.B8r.

"... his desires to have an heir to preserve his family name." Samuel Pepys, *The Diary of Samuel Pepys*, 1825 (Modern Library, 2001).

"... but he never became the father of a child." J. K. Amory, "George Washington's Infertility: Why Was the Father of Our Country Never a Father?" *Fertility and Sterility* 81, no. 3 (2004), 495–499.

"... the chances of his partner getting pregnant." Edmund S. S. Sabanegh Jr., ed., *Male Infertility: Problems and Solutions* (New York: Humana, 2010).

"... if something will be of help or harm to fertility." Bradley D Anawalt, "Diagnosis and Management of Anabolic Androgenic Steroid Use," *Journal of Clinical Endocrinology & Metabolism* 104, no. 7 (July 2019): 2490–2500.

"... obesity is linked to lower sperm counts and less fertility." Tod Fullston et al., "The Most Common Vices of Men Can Damage Fertility and the Health of the Next Generation," *Journal of Endocrinology*, 234, no. 2 (2017), F1–F6.

"... fruits, vegetables, and nuts to improve their fertility." Avicenna, *Ibn Sina's Canon of Medicine*, 1025 (Chicago: Kazi, 1999).

"... because they are all associated with decreased sperm counts." Feiby L. Nassan, Jorge E. Chavarro, and Cigdem Tanrikut, "Diet and Men's Fertility: Does Diet Affect Sperm Quality?" *Fertility and Sterility* 110, no. 4 (2018): 570–577.

"The creation of sperm is best achieved at 93°F (34°C)." Lidia Mínguez-Alarcón et al., "Type of Underwear Worn and Markers of Testicular Function among Men Attending a Fertility Center," *Human Reproduction* 33, no. 9 (2018), 1749–1756.

Chapter 4

"... removed from the *Diagnostic and Statistical Manual of Mental Disorders.*" Karen Stollznow, *On the Offensive: Prejudice in Language Past and Present* (Cambridge, UK: Cambridge University Press, 2020).

"... to treat joint pain such as arthritis and bursitis." James Harvey Young, *American Health Quackery* (Princeton, NJ: Princeton University Press, 2016).

"... Ulceration of the Womb, Irregularities, Floodings, etc." American Medical Association, *Female-Weakness Cures and Allied Frauds* (Chicago: Journal of the American Medical Association, 1915).

"... Pinkham's grandmotherly face was among the most recognizable in the world." Sarah Stage, *Female Complaints: Lydia Pinkham and the Business of Women's Medicine* (New York: W. W. Norton, 1981).

"... used by almost 90 percent of women who are trying to conceive." Edzard Ernst, "Herbal Medicinal Products during Pregnancy: Are They Safe?" *Obstetrics and Gynecology* 109, no. 3 (2002): 227–235.

"... Native American Algonquian language (... the plant's roots)." Cheryl Lans, Lisa Taylor-Swanson, and Rachel Westfall, "Herbal Fertility Treatments Used in North America from Colonial Times to 1900, and Their Potential for Improving the Success Rate of Assisted Reproductive Technology," *Reproductive Biomedicine & Society Online* 5 (2018): 60–81.

"... who were conceived after performing fertility rituals." Martha Ward, *Voodoo Queen: The Spirited Lives of Marie Laveau* (Jackson: University Press of Mississippi, 2004).

"... were often believed to have potent magical powers." Tony Kail, *A Secret History of Memphis Hoodoo: Rootworkers, Conjurers and Spirituals*, American Heritage (Charleston, SC: The History Press, 2017).

"... carved out of ebony by Baoulé people from the Côte d'Ivorie." "Lay Your Hands on the Legendary African Fertility Statues,"

Ripley's, accessed June 6, 2022, https://www.ripleys.com/fertility-statues/.

"... because she had neglected to also ask for childbirth." Nancy Demand, *Birth, Death, and Motherhood in Classical Greece* (Baltimore: Johns Hopkins University Press, 1994).

"... helped in delivery, and the barren to pregnancy." Plutarch, *Life of Julius Caesar* (Cambridge, MA: Loeb Classical Library, 1919).

"... was associated with a red gemstone." "The High Priest's Breastplate," Jewels for Me, accessed July 14, 2022, https://www.jewelsforme.com/gem_and_jewelry_library/curious_lore_chapter_eight#:~:text=According%20to%20the%20Rabbinical,Red.

"... burning desire for their translation into riches or other material objects." Napoleon Hill, *Think and Grow Rich*, rev. and exp. by Arthur R. Pell (New York: Tarcher Perigee, 2005; originally published 1937).

"... or render his sexual organs useless." Christopher Mackay, *The Hammer of Witches: A Complete Translation of the Malleus Maleficarum* (1486) (Cambridge, UK: Cambridge University Press, 2009).

"... was a result of being given the evil eye by an enemy." Dania H. Al-Jaroudi, "Beliefs of Subfertile Saudi Women," *Saudi Medical Journal* 31, no. 4 (2010): 425–427.

"... the reincarnation of Shiva, a Hindu god of fertility." Puja Changoiwala, "Prayed for a Child, Raped by a Godman: India's Deadly Childbirth Superstitions," *This Week in Asia*, October 5, 2018, https://www.scmp.com/week-asia/society/article/2165680/prayed-child-raped-godman-indias-deadly-childbirth-superstitions.

"... when alfalfa and soy were removed from her diet." Heather B. Patisaul, 2012. "Infertility in the Southern White Rhino: Is Diet the Source of the Problem?" *Endocrinology* 153, no. 4 (2012), 1568–1571.

"... including St. John's wort, echinacea, and gingko biloba." Glade B. Curtis and Judith Schuler, *Your Pregnancy Week by Week* (Philadelphia: DaCapo Lifelong, 2016).

"The Nirvana song 'Pennyroyal Tea' on the album *In Utero* is a reference to the popular use of the herb as an abortive aid." Nirvana, "Pennyroyal Tea," by Kurt Cobain, track 9 on *In Utero*, produced by Steve Albini, DGC Records, 1993.

". . . not intended to diagnose, treat, cure, or prevent any disease." Tracy A. Altman, *FDA and USDA Nutrition Labeling Guide: Decision Diagrams, Check* (Boca Raton, FL: CRC, 1998).

Chapter 5

". . . pregnancy for the first time at the age of 35 or older." George Uchenna Eleje et al., "Elderly Primigravidae versus Young Primigravidae: A Review of Pregnancy Outcome in a Low Resource Setting," *Nigerian Journal of Medicine* 23, no. 3 (2014): 220–229.

"Not only is there a biological clock for childbearing . . . 'Everybody's older. If you have somebody that's twenty-eight, it's like a teen pregnancy.'" F. C. Billari et al., "Social Age Deadlines for the Childbearing of Women and Men," *Human Reproduction* 26, no. 3 (2010): 616–622.

"The very first experimental laparoscopy was performed in 1901 on a live dog." Rosario Vecchio, B. V. MacFayden, and Francesco Palazzo, "History of Laparoscopic Surgery," *Panminerva Medica* 42, no. 1 (2000): 87–90.

". . . to try to diagnose infertility." Marten Stol, *Birth in Babylonia and the Bible: Its Mediterranean Setting* (Groningen: Styx, 2000), 33–37; Markham J. Geller, *Ancient Babylonian Medicine: Theory and Practice* (Chichester: Wiley-Blackwell, 2010).

"In his book . . . 'If you want to know . . . if not, she will not.'" Laurence Totelin, "Old Recipes, New Practice? The Latin Adaptations of the Hippocratic *Gynaecological Treatises*," *Social History of Medicine* 24, no. 1 (2011): 74–91.

"Hippocrates offers the following instructions: '. . . if not, she will not.'" Lois Magner and Oliver Kim, *A History of Medicine*, 3rd ed. (Boca Raton, FL: CRC, 2017).

"... older or are living with disabilities." "US Adoption Statistics," *Adoption Network*, accessed July 19, 2022, https://adoptionnetwork.com/adoption-myths-facts/domestic-us-statistics/.

"... normal and natural function of the body doesn't work the way it should." Victor Groza and Karen F. Rosenberg, *Clinical and Practice Issues in Adoption: Bridging the Gap between Adoptees Placed as Infants and as Older Children* (Westport, CT: Bergin & Garvey, 2001).

"... causing heartbreak for would-be parents." Taryn Hepburn et al., "'Their Reward Will Be a Lovely Daughter': The Mobilization of 'Hard to Adopt' and the Portrayal of Adoption as a Gift," *Adoption & Culture* 8, no. 2 (2020): 227–244.

"... a deep sense of loss, rejection, shame, guilt, and grief." David Brodzinsky, Megan Gunnar, and Jesús Palacios, "Adoption and Trauma: Risks, Recovery, and the Lived Experience of Adoption," *Child Abuse & Neglect*, September 17, 2021 (online ahead of print), doi: 10.1016/j.chiabu.2021.105309.

"... the 2.1 average needed to maintain a steady population." Brady E. Hamilton, Brady et al., "Births: Provisional Data for 2020," Division of Vital Statistics, National Center for Health Statistics, report no. 12 (May 2021), https://stacks.cdc.gov/view/cdc/104993.

"... and is linked to a decline in marriage." Gretchen Livingston, "Childlessness Falls, Family Size Grows among Highly Educated Women," Pew Research Center, May 7, 2015, https://www.pewresearch.org/social-trends/2015/05/07/childlessness-falls-family-size-grows-among-highly-educated-women/.

"... those who are at least planning to have them." Molly Ladd-Taylor and Lauri Umansky, eds., *"Bad" Mothers: The Politics of Blame in Twentieth-Century America* (New York: New York University Press, 1998).

"Oprah Winfrey ... adding, '... In fact, they overfill. I'm overflowed with maternal.'" "Here's Why Oprah Winfrey Refrains from Becoming a Mother!" *Business Standard*, October 11, 2019. https://www.business-standard.com/article/news-ani/

here-s-why-oprah-winfrey-refrains-from-becoming-a-mother-119101100463_1.html.

"... up to 20 percent suffer painful periods, or dysmenorrhea." Hong Ju, Mark Jones, and Gita Mishra, "The Prevalence and Risk Factors of Dysmenorrhea," *Epidemiologic Reviews* 36, no. 1 (2014): 104–113.

"Hippocrates came up with the concept of the 'wandering womb.'" Helen King, *Hippocrates' Women: Reading the Female Body in Ancient Greece* (Florence: Taylor & Francis, 2002).

"... causing health problems, including infertility." Philippe Morice et al., "History of Infertility," *Human Reproduction Update* 1, no. 5 (1995), 497–504.

"... too hot or humid: 'the great humidity ... she burns it and therefore she cannot conceive.'" Monica H. Green, ed., *The Trotula: An English Translation of the Medieval Compendium of Women's Medicine* (Philadelphia: University of Pennsylvania Press, 2002).

"... theory being that things which are too similar repel one another." Jennifer Evans, *Aphrodisiacs, Fertility and Medicine in Early Modern England* (Woodbridge, Suffolk: Royal Historical Society, Boydell, 2014).

"As the French physician Lazarus Riverius noted, for women, 'elderly years ... Conception.'" Sarah Toulalan, "'Elderly years cause a Total dispaire of Conception': Old Age, Sex and Infertility in Early Modern England," *Social History of Medicine* 29, no. 2 (2016), 333–359.

"In 1898, a doctor in Berlin wrote in the *German Journal of Physical Education*, '... strong children.'" Candice Goucher, *Women Who Changed the World: Their Lives, Challenges and Accomplishments throughout History*, 4 vols. (Santa Barbara, CA: ABC-CLIO, 2022).

"... something that arduous would make her uterus fall out." Katherine Switzer, *Marathon Woman: Running the Race to Revolutionize Women's Sports* (Boston: Da Capo, 2009).

"... inhibiting the development of the reproductive system." Edward H. Clarke, *Sex in Education; or, A Fair Chance for Girls* (Boston: James R. Osgood, 1873).

"... do indeed shrink after menopause." A. Lass and P. Brinsden, "The Role of Ovarian Volume in Reproductive Medicine," *Human Reproduction Update* 5, no. 3 (1999): 256–266.

"... which improves the chances of conception." Lamiya Mohiyiddeen et al., "Tubal Flushing for Subfertility," *Cochrane Database of Systematic Reviews* no. 5 (2015): CD003718.

"... significantly more likely to be the one to ovulate." I. Järvelä, S. Nuojua-Huttunen, and H. Martikainen, "Ovulation Side and Cycle Fecundity: A Retrospective Analysis of Frozen/Thawed Embryo Transfer Cycles," *Human Reproduction* 15, no. 6 (2000): 1247–1249.

Chapter 6

"And the doc went on to explain ... could find no purchase." Joel Coen and Etan Coen, *Raising Arizona*, directed by Joel Coen, Circle Films, 20th Century Fox, 1987.

"... Squire is described as 'a lover and lusty bacheler' ... chasing women." Geoffrey Chaucer, *The Canterbury Tales*, 1392 (London: Penguin Classics, 2003).

"... unprotected sex for one year or more." Sharon N. Covington and Linda Hammer Burns, eds., *Infertility Counseling: A Comprehensive Handbook for Clinicians*, 2nd ed. (Cambridge, UK: Cambridge University Press, 2006).

"... John Rock in Brookline, Massachusetts." Gayle Davis and Tracey Loughran, eds., *The Palgrave Handbook of Infertility in History* (London: Palgrave Macmillan, 2017).

"... individuals suffer from infertility worldwide." Kate O'Neill, "Opinion: Treating Infertility as a Disease," *The Scientist*, August 1, 2021, https://www.the-scientist.com/critic-at-large/opinion-treating-infertility-as-a-disease-68994.

"... any 'blockages,' but often causing infertility in the process."
Rebecca Flemming, "The Invention of Infertility in the Classical Greek World: Medicine, Divinity, and Gender," *Bulletin of
the History of Medicine* 87, no. 4 (2013), 565–590.

"... was also believed to benefit fertility." Jennifer Evans,
Aphrodisiacs, Fertility and Medicine in Early Modern England
(Woodbridge, Suffolk: Royal Historical Society, Boydell,
2014).

"... fathered at least twelve illegitimate children." Gary S. De Krey,
*Restoration and Revolution in Britain: Political Culture in the
Era of Charles II and the Glorious Revolution* (Basingstoke, NY:
Palgrave Macmillan, 2007).

"... which the film crew attributed to the 'fertility waters.'"
"Kidman Credits 'Fertility Waters' with Pregnancy," *Today*,
September 24, 2008, https://www.today.com/popculture/
kidman-credits-fertility-waters-pregnancy-1C9420900.

"... should try 'clove, spikenard, and nutmeg.'" Monica H. Green,
ed., *The Trotula: An English Translation of the Medieval Compendium of Women's Medicine* (Philadelphia: University of
Pennsylvania Press, 2002).

"... medical professionals don't recommend it." Jen Gunter,
"Gwyneth Paltrow Says Steam Your Vagina, an OB/GYN Says
Don't," *Dr. Jen Gunter*, January 27, 2015, https://drjengunter.
com/2015/01/27/gwyneth-paltrow-says-steam-your-vagina-
an-obgyn-says-dont/.

"Artificial insemination has a long history ... used by many world-
wide" W. Ombelet and J. Van Robays, "Artificial Insemination
History: Hurdles and Milestones," *Facts, Views & Vision in
ObGyn* 7, no. 2 (2015), 137–143.

"Birds have a more interesting reproductive system ... hens lay up
to three hundred eggs every year." Andy Cawthray and James
Hermes, *Chicken and Egg: An Egg-centric Guide to Raising
Poultry* (Lewes, UK: Ivy Press, 2015).

"... results in 15 percent per cycle." P. A. L. Kop et al., "Intrauterine Insemination or Intracervical Insemination with

Cryopreserved Donor Sperm in the Natural Cycle: A Cohort Study," *Human Reproduction* 30, no. 3 (2015): 603–607.

"... passes away, never having had any children." Pete Docter and Bob Peterson, *Up*, directed by Pete Docter, produced by Jonas Rivera, Walt Disney Pictures, Pixar Animation Studios, 2009.

"... the feel of a tiny hand that is never held?" Laura Bush, *Spoken from the Heart* (New York: Scribner, 2010).

"There is an apocryphal story about Ernest Hemingway... may have been inspired by a true story." "For sale: baby shoes, never worn," *Wikipedia*, last modified May 22, 2022, 07:20 (UTC), https://en.wikipedia.org/wiki/For_sale:_baby_shoes,_never_worn.

"In a 1910 edition of *The Spokane Press* ... 'This perhaps meant... sorrow and disappointment.'" "Tragedy of Baby's Death Is Revealed in Sale of Clothes," *The Spokane Press*, May 16, 1910, 6, https://commons.wikimedia.org/wiki/File:Babys_Clothes_Never_Worn.png.

"... biological clock." David E. Kelley, "Cro-Magnon," directed by Allan Arkush, *Ally McBeal*, season 1 (1998), episode 12.

"Infertility negatively affects quality of life and health, especially mental health." Alice D. Domar and Alice Lesch Kelly, *Conquering Infertility: Dr. Alice Domar's Mind/Body Guide to Enhancing Fertility and Coping with Infertility* (New York: Penguin, 2004).

"... frustrated, and worried all the time." A. D. Domar, P. C. Zuttermeister, and R. Friedman, "The Psychological Impact of Infertility: A Comparison with Patients with Other Medical Conditions," *Journal of Psychosomatic Obstetrics and Gynaecology* 14 Suppl (1993): 45–52.

"... but she's not actually expecting a baby." James Owen Drife, "Phantom Pregnancy," *British Medical Journal (Clinical Research Edition)* 291 (1985): 687.

"A famous example is that of Mary Tudor ... containing the 'Prayer for Expectant Mothers.'" Carolly Erickson, *Bloody Mary: The Life of Mary Tudor* (New York: St. Martin's Griffin, 1998).

"... then passes it off as her own." Michael Welner, Ann Burgess, and Kate O'Malley, "Psychiatric and Legal Considerations in Cases of Fetal Abduction by Maternal Evisceration," *Journal of Forensic Sciences* 66, no. 5 (2021): 1805–1817.

"... the implication being the happy ending that these were *their* children and grandchildren." Joel Coen and Etan Coen, *Raising Arizona*, directed by Joel Coen, Circle Films, 20th Century Fox, 1987.

Chapter 7

"... and on in vitro fertilization in rabbits." Margaret Marsh and Wanda Ronner, *The Pursuit of Parenthood: Reproductive Technology from Test-Tube Babies to Uterus Transplants* (Baltimore: Johns Hopkins University Press, 2019).

"... in endless rows of artificial wombs." Aldous Huxley, *Brave New World and Brave New World Revisited* (New York: Harper Perennial, 2005 [originally published in 1932]).

"... in which individuals were created outside of the human body." Vidyanand Nanjundiah, "J. B. S. Haldane: His Life and Science," *Current Science* 62, no. 9/10 (1992): 582–588.

"... but there were still many skeptics at the time." John Rock and Miriam F. Menkin, "In Vitro Fertilization and Cleavage of Human Ovarian Eggs," *Science* 100, no. 2588 (1944): 105–107.

"... first successful live birth of an IVF baby, Louise Joy Brown." Louise Brown and Martin Powell, *My Life as the World's First Test-Tube Baby* (Bristol: Bristol Books, 2015).

"... only 37.8 percent live births per embryo transfer." "ART Success Rates," Centers for Disease Control and Prevention, last reviewed March 17, 2022, https://www.cdc.gov/art/artdata/index.html.

"... economic disparities affect access to fertility treatments, especially IVF." Judith Daar et al., and the Ethics Committee of the American Society for Reproductive Medicine, "Disparities in Access to Effective Treatment for Infertility in the United

States: An Ethics Committee Opinion," *Fertility and Sterility* 104, no. 5 (2015): 1104–1110.

". . . following fifty-four years of marriage." India TV News Desk, "74-Year-Old Hyderabad Woman Creates History; Gives Birth to Healthy Twins," *India TV,* September 5, 2019, https:// www.indiatvnews.com/news/india-74-year-old-hyderabad- woman-gives-birth-twins-world-record-547490.

". . . fertility clinics in these countries are popular destinations for 'fertility tourism.'" Amy Speier, *Fertility Holidays: IVF Tourism and the Reproduction of Whiteness* (New York: New York University Press, 2016).

". . . in women who are "poor responders" to IVF stimulation medication." Francesco M. Fusi et al., "DHEA Supplementation Positively Affects Spontaneous Pregnancies in Women with Diminished Ovarian Function," *Gynecological Endocrinology* 29, no. 10 (2013): 940–943.

". . . by improving the quality of 'aging' eggs." Yilong Miao et al., "Nicotinamide Mononucleotide Supplementation Reverses the Declining Quality of Maternally Aged Oocytes," *Cell Reports* 32, no. 5 (2020): 107987.

". . . effective at improving egg quality and maturation." Asako Ochiai and Keiji Kuroda, "Preconception Resveratrol Intake against Infertility: Friend or Foe?" *Reproductive Medicine and Biology* 19, no. 2 (2019), 107–113.

". . . no firm evidence for their effectiveness in humans." Roger J. Hart, "Use of Growth Hormone in the IVF Treatment of Women with Poor Ovarian Reserve," *Frontiers in Endocrinology* 10 (2019): 500.

". . . the jury is still out on the matter." Ying C. Cheong et al., "Acupuncture and Assisted Reproductive Technology," *Cochrane Database of Systematic Reviews*, no. 7 (2013): CD006920.

". . . to use IVF to conceive their two daughters." Michelle Obama, *Becoming* (New York: Crown, 2018).

". . . who used IVF to conceive their children." BG Staff, "20 Celebs Who Had a Difficult Time Getting Pregnant,"

Babygaga, April 6, 2018, https://www.babygaga.
com/20-celebs-who-had-a-difficult-time-getting-pregnant/.

". . . He argued, 'The ultimate decision should be largely driven by the patient's wishes.'" Leslie Francis, ed., *The Oxford Handbook of Reproductive Ethics* (New York: Oxford University Press, 2017).

". . . used as a source of power." The Wachowski Brothers, *The Matrix*, directed by The Wachowskis, produced by Joel Silver, Warner Bros. et al., 1999.

". . . the best traits of their parents." Andrew Niccol, *Gattaca*, directed by Andrew Niccol, produced by Danny DeVito et al., Columbia Pictures, Jersey Films, Sony Pictures, 1997.

". . . a world where we have to consider the quality of our children." Susan Capel and Susan Piotrowski, eds., *Issues in Physical Education* (Milton Park, UK: Taylor & Francis, 2013).

". . . denounced IVF as 'playing God.'" Francis X. Rocca, "Pope Calls Abortion, Euthanasia, IVF Sins 'against God the Creator,'" *Catholic Register*, November 17, 2014, https://www.catholicregister.org/faith/item/19207-pope-calls-abortion-euthanasia-ivf-sins-against-god-the-creator.

"There are two main types of medication . . . (. . . postmenopausal nuns.)" Bruno Lunenfeld, "Gonadotropin stimulation: past, present and future," *Reprod Med Biol* 11, no. 1 (2011): 11–25.

". . . over-suppression, resulting in fewer follicles." J. Ou et al., "Short versus Long Gonadotropin-Releasing Hormone Analogue Suppression Protocols in IVF/ICSI Cycles in Patients of Various Age Ranges," *PLOS ONE* 10, no. 7 (2015): e0133887.

". . . laparoscopic surgery was used to collect the eggs." David K. Gardner and Carlos Simon, eds., *Handbook of In Vitro Fertilization*, 4th ed. (Boca Raton, FL: CRC Press, 2017).

". . . immediately after his death." Sophie Reardon, "Olympic Snowboarder's Widow Ellidy Pullin Welcomes Baby Girl via IVF 15 Months after His Death," *CBS News*, October 29, 2021, https://www.cbsnews.com/news/ellidy-pullin-baby-daughter-alex-chumpy-pullin-snowboarder-death-ivf/.

"... to form a new cell, called a zygote." Frank J. Longo, *Fertilization*, 2nd ed. (New York: Garland Science, 2020).

"... but to increase the profitability of the clinics that offer them." N. S. Macklon, K. K. Ahuja, and B. C. J. M. Fauser, "Building an Evidence Base for IVF 'Add-ons,'" *Reproductive Biomedicine* 38, no. 6 (2019): 853–856.

Conclusion

"... he writes, 'All parents want a little baby, and every child wants a little sister or brother.'" Hans Christian Andersen, "The Storks," tr. Jean Hersholt, *H. C. Andersen Centret*, accessed July 15, 2022, https://andersen.sdu.dk/vaerk/hersholt/TheStorks_e.html.

"... and empathy and healing which we so need." Web Desk, "Sharon Stone Shares Her Painful Story of Miscarriages, Says 'It Is No Small Thing,'" *The News*, June 24, 2022, https://www.thenews.com.pk/latest/968871-sharon-stone-shares-painful-story-of-miscarriages-says-it-is-no-small-thing.

"... still reminds her of her little brother." Dolly Parton and Porter Wagoner, vocalists, "Jeannie's Afraid of the Dark," written by Dolly Parton, track 3 on *Just the Two of Us*, RCA Records, 1968.

"... coming to accept her infertility and to embrace it." Dolly Parton and Robert K. Oermann, *Dolly Parton, Songteller: My Life in Lyrics* (San Francisco: Chronicle, 2020).

"... but now I realize that I am everybody's mother." Eryn Murphy, "Dolly Parton Once Explained to Andy Warhol Why She Never Had Children: 'I Tried for Years,'" *Showbiz CheatSheet*, January 7, 2022, https://www.cheatsheet.com/entertainment/dolly-parton-explained-andy-warhol-why-she-never-had-children-i-tried-for-years.html/.